Instructor's Guide for

Medical Terminology Simplified

A Programmed Learning Approach by Body System
Second Edition

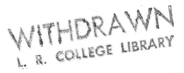
Barbara A. Gylys, MEd, CMA-A
Professor of Health and Human Services
Medical Assisting Technology
University of Toledo Community and Technical College
Toledo, Ohio

Regina M. Masters, BSN, RN, CMA, MEd
Instructor of Health and Human Services
University of Toledo Community and Technical College
Toledo, Ohio

 F. A. DAVIS COMPANY•Philadelphia

F. A. Davis Company
1915 Arch Street
Philadelphia, PA 19103

Last digit indicates print number: 10 9 8 7 6 5 4 3 2 1

Printed in the United States of America

0-8036-0346-0

CONTENTS

INTRODUCTION

The purpose of the *Instructor's Guide* is to help the teacher make the best possible use of the textbook and to provide a variety of supplemental teaching activities. The *Instructor's Guide* is organized according to the table of contents on pages iii–iv. Some of the special features include the following:

- Suggested course outlines
- Student outcomes and unit tests
- Medical reports with evaluations and dictionary exercises
- Anatomy coloring activities
- Crossword puzzles and solutions
- Master transparencies for each unit
- A CyberTest computerized test bank

The textbook and *Instructor's Guide* are designed to meet the criteria for competency-based education. Included are student outcomes for each unit that can be evaluated by written tests. The tests in the book and *Instructor's Guide* contain building words, fill-in blanks, words broken down into their component elements, and multiple-choice questions.

Achievement of minimal student scores, determined by individual instructors or institutions, will serve the function of meeting required competency standards. This technique provides not only flexibility in content but also the ability to tailor the course objectives according to the educational requirements of your institution.

The supplementary activities as well as the entire textbook can be used in either a classroom setting or as a self-instructional package. Included in each textbook are two audiocassette tapes that contain the pronunciations and definitions of medical words from each unit.

SUGGESTED COURSE OUTLINES

This textbook has been implemented in courses taught in various academic time frames and can be easily adapted to suit individual requirements. It is used successfully in traditional quarter and semester courses in orthodox college environments as well as in hospital-based curricula, insurance company classes, adult education courses, and proprietary school curricula.

The design of *Medical Terminology Simplified,* ed 2, permits a great deal of flexibilty, because each chapter can be self-tutorial or assigned as homework. The audiocassette tapes and availability of an interactive CD-ROM are provided to complement a self-paced approach.

Regardless of the academic time frame employed, it is important that Units 1 and 2 are covered first and thoroughly understood by the student. These two units provide the basic foundation of medical word building. Thereafter, selection of units as well as the extent of coverage presented is at the discretion of the individual teacher, although the authors recommend that the units be covered in sequential order. The criteria for competency-based curricula determine the content and scope of the course.

Sample course outlines for 10-week and 15-week classes are found in subsequent pages. These outlines are flexible and can be easily individualized to meet the curricular needs of various teaching institutions.

10-Week Course

Week 1,	**Day 1**	Unit 1 Introduction to Programmed Learning and Medical Word Building
	Day 2	Unit 2 Digestive System
Week 2,	**Day 1**	Unit 2 Digestive System
	Day 2	Unit 2 Digestive System
Week 3,	**Day 1**	Unit 3 Urinary System
	Day 2	Unit 3 Urinary System
Week 4,	**Day 1**	Unit 4 Integumentary System
	Day 2	Unit 5 Reproductive System
Week 5,	**Day 1**	Unit 5 Reproductive System
	Day 2	Unit 5 Reproductive System
Week 6,	**Day 1**	Unit 6 Respiratory System
	Day 2	Unit 6 Respiratory System
Week 7,	**Day 1**	Unit 7 Endocrine and Nervous Systems
	Day 2	Unit 7 Endocrine and Nervous Systems
Week 8,	**Day 1**	Unit 8 Musculoskeletal System
	Day 2	Unit 8 Musculoskeletal System
Week 9,	**Day 1**	Unit 9 Cardiovascular and Lymphatic Systems
	Day 2	Unit 9 Cardiovascular and Lymphatic Systems
Week 10,	**Day 1**	Unit 9 Cardiovascular and Lymphatic Systems
	Day 2	Unit 10 Special Senses: The Eyes and Ears

15-Week Course

Week 1,	**Day 1**	Unit 1 Introduction to Programmed Learning
	Day 2	Unit 2 Digestive System
Week 2,	**Day 1**	Unit 2 Digestive System
	Day 1	Unit 2 Digestive System
Week 3,	**Day 1**	Supplemental Activities from *Instructor's Guide*
	Day 2	Unit 3 Urinary System
Week 4,	**Day 1**	Unit 3 Urinary System
	Day 2	Unit 4 Integumentary System
Week 5,	**Day 1**	Supplemental Activities from *Instructor's Guide*
	Day 2	Unit 5 Reproductive System
Week 6,	**Day 1**	Unit 5 Reproductive System
	Day 2	Unit 5 Reproductive System
Week 7,	**Day 1**	Supplemental Activities from *Instructor's Guide*
	Day 2	Review for Mid-semester Exam
Week 8,	**Day 1**	Unit 6 Respiratory System
	Day 2	Unit 6 Respiratory System
Week 9,	**Day 1**	Unit 7 Endocrine and Nervous Systems
	Day 2	Unit 7 Endocrine and Nervous Systems
Week 10,	**Day 1**	Supplemental Activities from *Instructor's Guide*
	Day 2	Unit 8 Musculoskeletal System
Week 11,	**Day 1**	Unit 8 Musculoskeletal System
	Day 2	Supplemental Activities from the *Instructor's Guide*
Week 12,	**Day 1**	Unit 9 Cardiovascular and Lymphatic Systems
		Unit 9 Cardiovascular and Lymphatic Systems
Week 13,	**Day 1**	Unit 9 Cardiovascular and Lymphatic Systems
	Day 2	Supplemental Activities from *Instructor's Guide*
Week 14,	**Day 1**	Special Senses: The Eyes and Ears
	Day 2	Special Senses: The Eyes and Ears

DISTANCE LEARNING

As we prepare to enter the new millennium, the computer revolution in education is exerting an increasing influence on teachers and students at all levels of education. Educators are being challenged to integrate the latest technology into the learning process in order to promote a commitment to excellence in education and a high level of performance among future professionals. New alternative learning systems are being developed to meet students' needs, one of which is distance learning. This type of education is delivered to remote sites through technology such as two-way video, cablevision, the Internet, and e-mail. It is a means of providing educational access to students who otherwise would not have it. Some see it as a continuing education tool for those who are gainfully employed and need to keep updated. Educational institutions have recognized that this technology can provide entrepreneurial opportunities for universities and colleges all over the world. Current distance learning websites include general information about courses, course requirements, course syllabi, interactive chat rooms with bulletin board–type discussions, and direct e-mail access between instructors and/or students enrolled in the courses. The distance learning technology available at your school or institution will determine the sophistication of implementing the latest technological teaching tools.

To help instructors design a medical terminology course with ancillary teaching aids that complements a distance learning course, the authors have provided a variety of teaching aids, including an *Interactive Medical Terminology CD-ROM* program that is designed at a 90 percent competency level. Descriptions and illustrations of the entire learning package for *Medical Terminology Simplified* are presented below.

Audiocassette Tapes. Two audiocassette tapes are included with each textbook. Medical terms covered in a body system's unit are summarized at the end of the unit and identified with the corresponding frames from which they originate. Thus, additional information can be obtained and reviewed as the pronunciations of the terms are given on the audiocassette tape.

Interactive CD-ROM. The instructor may choose to adopt the book with a multimedia *Interactive Medical Terminology CD-ROM.* This competency-based software is self-paced and includes graphics, voice, a dictionary, help menus, printouts of a student's progress, along with numerous activities that are designed at a 90% competency level.

UNIT 1 INTRODUCTION TO PROGRAMMED LEARNING AND MEDICAL WORD BUILDING

STUDENT OUTCOMES

Upon completion of this unit, you will be able to:

◆ Define and provide several examples of word roots, combining forms, and suffixes.

◆ Divide medical words into component parts.

◆ Describe how medical words are formed from word roots, combining forms, and suffixes, and apply this knowledge by completing the review exercises.

Unit 1 Introduction to Programmed Learning and Medical Word Building

Multiple choice: Select the best answer.

1. Which suffix is an adjective ending?
    a. -oma
    b. -penia
    a. -itis
    a. -ic
    b. -ia

Answer: d

2. The word that contains a prefix is
    a. implant
    b. planting
    c. planter
    d. planted
    e. plant

Answer: a

3. A combining form is a word root plus a
    a. prefix
    b. vowel
    c. suffix
    d. another word root
    e. consonant

Answer: b

4. The combining form gastr/o refers to the
    a. mouth
    b. intestine
    c. stomach
    d. liver
    e. bladder

Answer: c

5. The suffix -itis means
   a. pain
   b. blood
   c. excision
   d. rupture
   e. inflammation

Answer: e

6. Which of the following is NOT a combining form?
   a. gastr/o
   b. arthr/o
   c. angi
   d. nephr/o
   e. mast/o

Answer: c

7. A word root usually indicates a
   a. position
   b. number
   c. condition
   d. body part
   e. procedure

Answer: d

8. An element located at the beginning of a medical word is a
   a. prefix
   b. suffix
   c. combining vowel
   d. a and c
   e. b and c

Answer: a

9. In the word therm/o/meter, -meter is
   a. an adjective
   b. a prefix
   c. a combining form
   d. a compound word
   e. a suffix

Answer: e

10. Arthr/o/centesis means puncture of a joint. In this word, arthr/o is a
    a. prefix
    b. suffix
    c. word root
    d. combining vowel
    e. combining form

Answer: e

11. When building a medical word, a combining form is used before a suffix that begins with a
    a. prefix
    b. suffix
    c. vowel
    d. consonant
    e. letter "o"

Answer: d

12. Which of the following words is built INCORRECTLY?
    a. my/algia
    b. nephr/o/dynia
    c. aden/oid
    d. gastr/plasty
    e. py/o/rrhea

Answer: d

13. Which of the following is a word root?
    a. hepat
    b. hepato
    c. hepatom
    d. -megaly
    e. hepatomegaly

Answer: a

14. Which of the following is an example of a combining form that is used to link one word root to another word root?
    a. gastr/itis
    b. gastr/o/dynia
    c. gastr/o/esophag/itis
    d. gastr/o/megaly
    e. gastr/oma

Answer: c

15. The prefix in post/mortem means
    a. before
    b. after
    c. death
    d. life
    e. beyond

Answer: b

UNIT 2   DIGESTIVE SYSTEM

STUDENT OUTCOMES

Upon completion of this unit, you will be able to:

♦ Explain the main functions of the digestive system.

♦ Identify the organs of the alimentary canal.

♦ Identify the accessory organs of digestion.

♦ Explain the role of the liver and gallbladder in digestion.

♦ Identify the combining forms and suffixes related to the organs and structures of the digestive system.

♦ Build and analyze medical terms related to the digestive system by completing the frames and reviews.

♦ Identify pathology related to the digestive system.

♦ Evaluate medical reports.

♦ Spell and pronounce medical terms by completing the audiocassette activities.

Unit 2 Digestive System

Multiple choice: Select the best answer.

1. A condition in which there is excessive flow of saliva is known as
   a. gastr/o/rrhea
   b. sial/o/rrhea
   c. dia/rrhea
   d. chol/emesis
   e. hyper/emesis

Answer: b

2. Bleeding of the gums is a primary symptom of
   a. gingiv/itis
   b. sial/itis
   c. esophag/itis
   d. stomat/itis
   e. peri/odont/itis

Answer: a

3. The mechanical process of digestion begins in the
   a. mouth
   b. esophagus
   c. stomach
   d. small intestine
   e. large intestine

Answer: a

4. Which of the following diseases could result from contact with infected blood?
   a. Crohn's disease
   b. pancreatitis
   c. hematemesis
   d. hepatitis B
   e. mycosis

Answer: d

5. Which of the following specialist(s) is CORRECTLY matched with the procedure(s) performed?
   a. periodontist—straightens teeth
   b. gastrologist—treats gingivitis
   c. cardiologist—treats heart disease
   d. orthodontist—treats tooth pain
   e. all of the above are correctly matched

Answer: c

6. A chole/lith is a
   a. pancreatic stone
   b. liver stone
   c. salivary stone
   d. gallstone
   e. stomach stone

Answer: d

7. Which of the following statements regarding anatomic positions is TRUE?
   a. The esophagus is inferior to the stomach.
   b. The stomach is superior to the duodenum.
   c. The rectum is inferior to the anus.
   d. The jejunum is inferior to the ileum.
   e. The duodenum is inferior to the jejunum.

Answer: b

8. The term lingu/o/gingiv/al means pertaining to
   a. the tongue and salivary glands
   b. the salivary glands and the gums
   c. the teeth and the tongue
   d. the tongue and the gums
   e. the teeth and the gums

Answer: d

9. A gastr/o/scopy is performed with
   a. a gastrotome
   b. a fiberoptic tube
   c. a gastrotomy
   d. x-ray equipment
   e. an esophagotome

Answer: b

10. Dys/phagia results from a problem with the
    a. esophagus
    b. stomach
    c. small intestine
    d. colon
    e. rectum

Answer: a

11. Which of the following pairs of glands or organs is INCORRECTLY matched with its secretion?
    a. parotid gland—saliva
    b. pancreas—insulin
    c. liver—bile
    d. gallbladder—chyme
    e. stomach—gastric juices

Answer: d

12. Crohn's disease is a chronic infection of the
    a. rectum
    b. esophagus
    c. anus
    d. stomach
    e. ileum

Answer: e

13. Which of the following is a surgical procedure?
    a. cholecystography
    b. hepatectomy
    c. sigmoidoscope
    d. gastrorrhea
    e. proctodynia

Answer: b

14. A person usually takes antacids to obtain relief from
    a. aerophagia
    b. stomatitis
    c. dyspepsia
    d. sialitis
    e. diarrhea

Answer: c

15. The medical term for excision of the small intestine is
    a. gastrectomy
    b. colectomy
    c. enterorrhaphy
    d. enterectomy
    e. colorrhaphy

Answer: d

16. A visual examination of the rectum and anus is a(n)
    a. sigmoidoscopy
    b. colonoscopy
    c. enteroscopy
    d. coloscopy
    e. proctoscopy

Answer: e

17. A bleeding duodenal ulcer would most likely result in
    a. diarrhea
    b. sialorrhea
    c. hyperemesis
    d. cholemesis
    e. hematemesis

Answer: e

18. During digestion, the bile ducts pass gall from the gallbladder to the
    a. stomach
    b. small intestine
    c. colon
    d. liver
    e. pancreas

Answer: b

19. Bile is produced by the
    a. stomach
    b. salivary glands
    c. pancreas
    d. liver
    e. gallbladder

Answer: d

20. Which of the following is NOT part of the small intestine?
    a. cecum
    b. ileum
    c. duodenum
    d. jejunum
    e. all of the above are part of the small intestine

Answer: a

21. The pear-shaped, saclike organ that serves as a reservoir for bile is the
    a. liver
    b. pancreas
    c. gallbladder
    d. spleen
    e. duodenum

Answer: c

22. All of the following are salivary glands EXCEPT
    a. sublingual
    b. submandibular
    c. submaxillary
    d. lingual
    e. parotid

Answer: d

23. The medical term that means a stricture or narrowing of the rectum is
    a. rectodynia
    b. rectoplasty
    c. rectospasm
    d. rectopexy
    e. rectostenosis

Answer: e

24. The following are parts of the colon EXCEPT
    a. ascending
    b. descending
    c. sigmoid
    d. transverse
    e. all of the above are parts of the colon

Answer: e

25. A visual examination of the sigmoid colon is
    a. sigmoidoscope
    b. sigmoidoscopy
    c. sigmoidotomy
    d. sigmoidostomy
    e. sigmoidopexy

Answer: b

26. Binging and purging are also known as
    a. anorexia
    b. hematemesis
    c. bulimia
    d. dysphagia
    e. anorexia nervosa

Answer: c

27. Protrusion of an organ through a wall is known as
    a. a reflux
    b. a perforation
    c. a volvulus
    d. diverticulosis
    e. a hernia

Answer: e

28. The medical word for accumulation of serous fluids in the abdominal cavity is
    a. flatus
    b. anorexia
    c. ascites
    d. bulimia
    e. edema

Answer: c

29. A life-threatening obstruction in which the bowel twists upon itself is
    a. intussusception
    b. a volvulus
    c. peritonitis
    d. ischemia
    e. a hernia

Answer: b

30. Crohn's disease is a bowel disorder that is also known as
    a. diarrhea
    b. volvulus
    c. ischemia
    d. melena
    e. regional ileitis

Answer: e

UNIT 3   URINARY SYSTEM

STUDENT OUTCOMES

Upon completion of this unit, you will be able to:

♦ Explain the main functions of the urinary system.

♦ Identify the organs of the urinary system.

♦ Identify the combining forms and suffixes related to the organs and structures of the urinary system.

♦ Build and analyze medical terms related to the urinary system by completing the frames and reviews.

♦ Identify pathology related to the urinary system.

♦ Evaluate medical reports.

♦ Spell and pronounce medical terms by completing the audiocassette activities.

Unit 3: Urinary System

Multiple choice: Select the best answer.

1. Bright's disease is another name for
   a. urethritis
   b. ureteralgia
   c. cystitis
   d. glomerulonephritis
   e. pyelopathy

Answer: d

2. The crushing of a stone is called
   a. lithotomy
   b. lithotripsy
   c. lithectomy
   d. lithiasis
   e. lithoscope

Answer: b

3. In nephrorrhaphy there is
   a. hemorrhage in the kidney
   b. a stone present in the kidney
   c. an inflammation of the kidney
   d. a prolapse of the kidney
   e. suturing of the kidney

Answer: e

4. The act of voiding urine is called
   a. nocturia
   b. micturition
   c. oliguria
   d. urodynia
   e. pyorrhea

Answer: b

5. The initials UTI stand for
   a. urethral toxic infection
   b. ureter total inflammation
   c. urinary tract incontinence
   d. urinary tract infection
   e. ureter tubal infection

Answer: d

6. Which of the following sets of terms have the same meaning?
   a. cystitis—pyelitis
   b. urethrodynia—urethralgia
   c. oliguria—anuria
   d. nephritis—nephrosis
   e. leukocyte—leukorrhea

Answer: b

7. Adenodynia is pain in
   a. the intestines
   b. the stomach
   c. a gland
   d. the pelvic area
   e. the gallbladder

Answer: c

8. A ureterolith would be found
   a. in the tubules of the nephron
   b. in the tube between the kidneys and the bladder
   c. in the bladder
   d. in the renal pelvis
   e. in the canal extending from the bladder to outside the body

Answer: b

9. Cystectomy is the medical term for
   a. an incision into the bladder
   b. excision of the bladder
   c. incision into the kidney
   d. excision of the kidney
   e. creation of a new opening in the kidney

Answer: b

10. A urotoxin is
    a. a poison in the ureter
    b. a poison in the urethra
    c. a poison in the urine
    d. the study of poisons
    e. a red substance in the urine

Answer: c

11. A patient with a stone in the ureter would most likely experience
    a. ureterodynia
    b. nocturia
    c. polyuria
    d. cystitis
    e. homeostasis

Answer: a

12. A suprarenal tumor is located
    a. within the kidney
    b. under the kidney
    c. upon the kidney
    d. within the bladder
    e. upon the bladder

Answer: c

13. Which of the following terms means increased urinary production?
   a. oliguria
   b. polyuria
   c. anuria
   d. micturition
   e. continence

Answer: b

14. The surgical procedure to correct a prolapsed kidney is termed
   a. nephroptosis
   b. nephrodesis
   c. nephrotomy
   d. nephropexy
   e. nephrostomy

Answer: d

15. The urinary tract is composed of the
   a. vagina, urethra, and bladder
   b. ureters, bladder, and cervix
   c. kidneys, ureters, and bladder
   d. prostate, bladder, and urethra
   e. kidneys, colon, and bladder

Answer: c

16. The ureters carry urine from the kidneys to the
   a. urethra
   b. bladder
   c. renal pelvis
   d. renal artery
   e. meatus

Answer: b

17. The medical word for scanty urinary output is
    a. icturia
    b. oliguria
    c. uremia
    d. hematuria
    e. polyuria

Answer: b

18. Uncontrolled loss of urine from the bladder is
    a. continence
    b. incontinence
    c. urination
    d. nocturia
    e. anuria

Answer: b

19. The abbreviation for intravenous pyelogram is
    a. IP
    b. INP
    c. IPG
    d. IVPG
    e. IVP

Answer: e

20. Agents that promote the secretion of urine are
    a. uremics
    b. antidiuretics
    c. diaphoretics
    d. uricosurics
    e. diuretics

Answer: e

21. The microscopic filtering units responsible for maintaining homeostasis are
    a. calyces
    b. nephrons
    c. collecting tubules
    d. Bowman's capsules
    e. ureters

Answer: b

22. An excessive amount of fluid contained within body tissues is called
    a. diuretic
    b. lithiasis
    c. cystitis
    d. edema
    e. hematuria

Answer: d

23. The funnel-shaped reservoir that is the basin of the kidney is the
    a. renal pelvis
    b. calyces
    c. urethra
    d. nephron
    e. bladder

Answer: a

24. The instrument used for a cystoscopy is a
    a. cystotome
    b. cystitis
    c. cystoscope
    d. cystectomy
    e. cystostomy

Answer: c

25. Herniation of the urethra is termed a
    a. rectocele
    b. ureterocele
    c. pyelopathy
    d. urethrocele
    e. nephritis

Answer: d

26. An abnormal congenital opening of the male urethra upon the undersurface of the penis is a(n)
    a. phimosis
    b. epididymitis
    c. uremia
    d. cryptorchidism
    e. hypospadias

Answer: e

27. Painful urination is known as
    a. anuria
    b. polyuria
    c. dysuria
    d. nocturia
    e. hematuria

Answer: c

28. An increase in nitrogenous compounds in urine is
    a. azotemia
    b. polyuria
    c. enuresis
    d. dysuria
    e. uremia

Answer: a

29. Stenosis of the foreskin opening over the glans penis is
    a. hypospadias
    b. interstitial nephritis
    c. phimosis
    d. uremia
    e. Wilm's tumor

Answer: c

30. Urinary incontinence such as bedwetting is
    a. enuresis
    b. diuresis
    c. oliguria
    d. hemoptysis
    e. hyperuricemia

Answer: a

UNIT 4   INTEGUMENTARY SYSTEM

STUDENT OUTCOMES

Upon completion of this unit, you will be able to:

♦ Explain the purpose of the integumentary system.

♦ Identify the structures of the integumentary system.

♦ Identify the combining forms and suffixes related to the structures of the integumentary system.

♦ Build and analyze medical terms related to the integumentary system by completing the frames and reviews.

♦ Identify pathology related to the respiratory system.

♦ Analyze medical reports.

♦ Spell and pronounce medical terms by completing the audiocassette activities.

Unit 4: Integumentary System

Multiple choice: Select the best answer.

1. Cyanosis of the skin will result from
    a. excessive sun exposure
    b. increased levels of blood cholesterol
    c. insufficient leukocytes in the blood
    d. excessive dryness of the skin
    e. insufficient oxygen in the blood

Answer: e

2. Which of the following cells are found in the blood?
    a. erythrocytes
    b. melanocytes
    c. xanthocytes
    d. lipocytes
    e. histiocytes

Answer: a

3. A person with trichopathy has a disease of the
    a. sweat glands
    b. fingernails
    c. skin
    d. hair
    e. stomach

Answer: d

4. A person who has psoriasis will experience
    a. syncope
    b. cyanosis
    c. colitis
    d. hidrosis
    e. pruritus

Answer: e

5. Which of the following words is paired with the correct definition?
   a. leukemia—decrease in white blood cells
   b. onychoma—hernia of nail bed
   c. syncope—fainting
   d. sclerosis—softening
   e. vulgaris—rare

Answer: c

6. The disease that results when the body is not producing insulin is
   a. psoriasis
   b. enteritis
   c. hidrorrhea
   d. onychopathy
   e. diabetes mellitus

Answer: e

7. Overfunctioning sudoriferous glands produce excessive amounts of
   a. oil
   b. sweat
   c. insulin
   d. fat
   e. white blood cells

Answer: b

8. Which of the following conditions would be treated by a dermatologist?
   a. skin disorders
   b. sinus problems
   c. blood disorders
   d. stomach disorders
   e. diabetes mellitus

Answer: a

9. A person with sunburn will have
   a. xanthoderma
   b. melanoderma
   c. erythroderma
   d. cyanosis
   e. scleroderma

Answer: c

10. In scleroderma, the skin is
    a. hardened
    b. blue
    c. enlarged
    d. softened
    e. black

Answer: a

11. A dermatome is an
    a. instrument used to remove fat cells
    b. instrument used to cut the skin
    c. an incision made into the skin
    d. a and b
    e. a and c

Answer: b

12. The medical history of a patient indicates he has pruritus of the hands. This means the patient has
    a. excessive sweating of the hands
    b. a disease of the nails of the hand
    c. an inflammation of the hands
    d. itching of the hands
    e. a skin condition that turns the hands blue

Answer: d

13. Which of the following terms are synonyms?
    a. hidrosis—hidrorrhea
    b. adipectomy—adenectomy
    c. adenoma—onychoma
    d. xeroderma—scleroderma
    e. leukemia—leukocytopenia

Answer: a

14. A condition of yellow skin is
   a. xanthoderma
   b. xeroderma
   c. scleroderma
   d. melanoderma
   e. erythroderma

Answer: a

15. A malignant black tumor of the skin is
   a. an onychoma
   b. a xanthoma
   c. an adenoma
   d. a hidradenoma
   e. a melanoma

Answer: e

16. When a person's white blood cell count is below normal, the person's condition is called
   a. leukemia
   b. xanthemia
   c. leukocytopenia
   d. xanthosis
   e. leukoderma

Answer: c

17. Which of the following conditions results from skin deposits of excess levels of blood cholesterol?
   a. adipocele
   b. histiocytoma
   c. melanosis
   d. xanthomas
   e. psoriasis

Answer: d

18. A lack of pigmentation in the skin results in a condition called
    a. erythroderma
    b. cyanoderma
    c. leukoderma
    d. xanthoderma
    e. xeroderma

Answer: c

19. Dermatitis is the medical term for
    a. darkening of the skin
    b. inflammation of the skin
    c. dryness of the skin
    d. hardening of the skin
    e. itching of the skin

Answer: b

20. The layer of loose connective tissue that lies beneath the dermis is the
    a. adipose
    b. subcutaneous
    c. superficial
    d. vascular
    e. muscular

Answer: b

21. A tumor of the nail (or nailbed) is known as
    a. lipoma
    b. adenoma
    c. onychoma
    d. melanoma
    e. adipoma

Answer: c

22. The medical term for warts, moles, and pimples is
    a. macules
    b. papules
    c. xanthomas
    d. xerodermas
    e. lipomas

Answer: b

23. Excessive dryness of skin is called
    a. hidrosis
    b. leukoderma
    c. scleroderma
    d. xeroderma
    e. xerophagia

Answer: d

24. A physician who specializes in skin diseases is a(n)
    a. gastrologist
    b. oncologist
    c. hematologist
    d. gynecologist
    e. dermatologist

Answer: e

25. The chronic skin disease that is usually marked by itchy, scaly, red patches covered by silvery gray scales is
    a. vulgaris
    b. melanoma
    c. xeroderma
    d. psoriasis
    e. erythema

Answer: d

26. An inflammatory skin disease characterized by isolated pustules that become crusted and rupture is
    a. hirsutism
    b. pemphigus
    c. impetigo
    d. eczema
    e. psoriasis

Answer: c

27. Localized loss of skin pigmentation is
    a. tinea
    b. scabies
    c. purpura
    d. ecchymosis
    e. vitiligo

Answer: e

28. Another term for a blackhead is
    a. melanoma
    b. chloasma
    c. pemphigus
    d. petechia
    e. comedo

Answer: e

29. Fungal skin disease is called
    a. tinea
    b. pemphigus
    c. eczema
    d. vulgaris
    e. ecchymosis

Answer: a

30. A contagious skin disease transmitted by the itch mite is
    a. melanoma
    b. trichopathy
    c. scabies
    d. abrasion
    e. psoriasis

Answer: c

UNIT 5   REPRODUCTIVE SYSTEM

STUDENT OUTCOMES

Upon completion of this unit, you will be able to do:

♦ Explain the main functions of the reproductive system.

♦ Identify the organs of the reproductive system.

♦ Identify the combining forms and suffixes related to the organs and structures of the reproductive system.

♦ Build and analyze medical terms related to the reproductive system by completing the frames and reviews.

♦ Identify pathology related to the respiratory system.

♦ Evaluate medical reports.

♦ Sell and pronounce medical terms by completing the audiocassette activities.

Unit 5: Reproductive System

Multiple choice: Select the best answer.

1. The structure that transports sperm from the testes to the urethra
   a. prostate gland
   b. testes
   c. epididymis
   d. vas deferens
   e. seminal vesicles

Answer: d

2. A hernia of the fallopian tube is called a
   a. hysterocele
   b. colpocystocele
   c. salpingocele
   d. hydrocele
   e. metrocele

Answer: c

3. A woman with colpodynia is suffering from pain in the
   a. ovary
   b. fallopian tube
   c. cervix
   d. uterus
   e. vagina

Answer: e

4. The neck of the uterus is called the
   a. labia minora
   b. vulva
   c. clitoris
   d. cervix
   e. Bartholin's gland

Answer: d

5. Another term for Cowper's glands is
   a. prostate
   b. bulbourethral
   c. Bartholin's
   d. epididymis
   e. testes

Answer: b

6. Which organ surrounds the neck of the bladder and the urethra in a male?
   a. epididymis
   b. prostate gland
   c. testes
   d. Cowper's glands
   e. vas deferens

Answer: b

7. An orchidorrhaphy is
   a. the rupture of an ovary
   b. hemorrhage of the vagina
   c. the suture of a testicle
   d. the fixation of an ovary
   e. a discharge from a testicle

Answer: c

8. A medical term meaning inflammation of the uterus is
   a. hysteritis
   b. salpingitis
   c. colpitis
   d. mastitis
   e. vaginitis

Answer: a

9. Testosterone is produced by the
   a. ovaries
   b. testes
   c. uterus
   d. prostate
   e. epididymis

Answer: b

10. Progesterone is secreted by the
    a. ovaries
    b. uterus
    c. fallopian tubes
    d. testes
    e. prostate

Answer: a

11. The female external genitalia include each of the following structures EXCEPT
    a. the vagina
    b. Bartholin's glands
    c. the labia majora
    d. the labia minora
    e. the clitoris

Answer: a

12. When menstruation ceases permanently as a result of the aging process, it is called
    a. menorrhagia
    b. metrorrhagia
    c. menopause
    d. amenorrhea
    e. amenorrhagia

Answer: c

13. The notation "gravida 2, para 1" denotes a woman who has had
    a. pregnancy and 2 live births
    b. 2 pregnancies and 1 live birth
    c. 2 pregnancies and 1 miscarriage
    d. 2 pregnancies and 1 abortion
    e. 2 pregnancies and 1 stillbirth

Answer: b

14. A PID is the abbreviation for
    a. progesterone-induced dysmenorrhea
    b. prenatal infectious disease
    c. pelvic inflammatory dysplasia
    d. postmenopausal-induced disorder
    e. pelvic inflammatory disease

Answer: e

15. Which of the following terms are synonyms?
    a. salpingitis—oophoritis
    b. metritis—hysteritis
    c. colpitis—cervicitis
    d. vaginitis—vulvitis
    e. all are synonyms

Answer: b

16. The term postnatal means
    a. happening before birth
    b. happening after birth
    c. happening before conception
    d. happening after conception
    e. happening after menopause

Answer: b

17. In salpingitis, which of the following structures is affected?
    a. ovaries
    b. vagina
    c. uterus
    d. cervix
    e. fallopian tubes

Answer: e

18. Metropathy is a term for a disease of the
    a. ovaries
    b. fallopian tubes
    c. breasts
    d. uterus
    e. vagina

Answer: d

19. The term colpocervical refers to the
    a. uterus and cervix
    b. vagina and uterus
    c. ovary and uterus
    d. vagina and cervix
    e. fallopian tubes and cervix

Answer: d

20. An excessive increase in the number of cells in a tissue or organ
    a. a hydrocele
    b. a hematoma
    c. hyperplasia
    d. an adipoid
    e. hypertrophy

Answer: c

21. Each of the following pairs of words are synonyms EXCEPT
    a. adipoid—lipoid
    b. colpodynia—vasalgia
    c. testes—testicles
    d. menses—menstruation
    e. mammary gland—breast

Answer: b

22. Hesitancy, dysuria, hematuria, and frequency are symptoms of
    a. hydronephrosis
    b. prostatic carcinoma
    c. glomerulitis
    d. hydrocele
    e. varicocele

Answer: b

23. Enlargement of the prostate gland is termed
    a. prostatomegaly
    b. prostatitis
    c. prostatectomy
    d. prostatalgia
    e. prostatorrhea

Answer: a

24. An instrument used for examining the vagina and cervix uteri is a
    a. colposcopy
    b. colposcope
    c. salpingoscopy
    d. salpingoscope
    e. cystoscope

Answer: b

25. The abbreviation that indicates instrumental expansion of the cervix and
    scraping of the uterine cavity is
    a. C&S
    b. E&S
    c. D&C
    d. IUD
    e. PID

Answer: c

26. Benign prostatic hyperplasia
    a. is associated with the female reproductive system
    b. is associated with the male reproductive system
    c. is common in young adults
    d. may obstruct urinary flow
    e. b and d

Answer: e

27. The surgical procedure that sterilizes the male and prevents the release of sperm is
    a. prostatectomy
    b. vasectomy
    c. orchiorrhaphy
    d. hysterectomy
    e. testopathy

Answer: b

28. The condition of improperly descended testicles is referred to as
    a. orchiopexy
    b. varicocele
    c. ectopy of the testicle
    d. hydrocele
    e. cryptorchidism

Answer: e

29. The primary sore of syphilis is a
    a. chancre
    b. chlamydia
    c. herpes
    d. trichomoniasis
    e. moniliasis

Answer: a

30. The discharge associated with candidiasis is
    a. yellowish
    b. frothy
    c. curdy
    d. bloody
    e. clear

Answer: a

UNIT 6   RESPIRATORY SYSTEM

STUDENT OUTCOMES

Upon completion of this unit, you will be able to:

◆ Explain the main functions of the respiratory system.

◆ Identify the organs and structures of the respiratory system.

◆ Identify the combining forms and suffixes related to the organs and structures of the respiratory system.

◆ Build and analyze medical terms related to the respiratory system by completing the frames and reviews.

◆ Identify pathology related to the respiratory system.

◆ Evaluate medical reports.

◆ Spell and pronounce medical terms by completing the audiocassette activities.

Unit 6: Respiratory System

Multiple choice: Select the best answer.

1. Which of the following words is a plural form?
   a. bronchus
   b. alveolus
   c. fungus
   d. nares
   e. polyp

Answer: d

2. The natural process of drawing air into the lungs is called
   a. aerotherapy
   b. aspiration
   c. expiration
   d. orthopnea
   e. inspiration

Answer: e

3. A lobectomy is a procedure that removes a portion of the
   a. larynx
   b. diaphragm
   c. lung
   d. nose
   e. trachea

Answer: c

4. A nosebleed is known as
   a. ascites
   b. anoxia
   c. anosmia
   d. epistaxis
   e. empyema

Answer: d

5. A narrowing or stricture of the voice box is called
   a. pharyngostenosis
   b. laryngostenosis
   c. pneumostenosis
   d. laryngospasm
   e. pharyngospasm

Answer: b

6. During the swallowing process, the structure that closes off the larynx
   is the
   a. pharynx
   b. epiglottis
   c. fascia
   d. trachea
   e. septum

Answer: b

7. The following sets of words are synonyms EXCEPT
   a. trachea—windpipe
   b. larynx—voice box
   c. pharynx—throat
   d. necropsy—biopsy
   e. nares—nostrils

Answer: d

8. A chondroma is a tumor composed of
   a. muscle
   b. bone
   c. liver cells
   d. lung tissue
   e. cartilage

Answer: e

9. When a person has difficulty breathing when not in a sitting or standing position, the person's condition is known as
   a. dyspnea
   b. orthopnea
   c. apnea
   d. eupnea
   e. aerophagia

Answer: b

10. A medical term for involuntary contractions of the bronchi is
    a. bronchiectasis
    b. bronchospasm
    c. bronchostenosis
    d. bronchorrhagia
    e. bronchitis

Answer: b

11. A medical term meaning pain in the double membrane that covers the lungs is
    a. bronchiectasis
    b. pleuralgia
    c. pneumonomalacia
    d. pharyngoplegia
    e. pneumonopathy

Answer: b

12. The medical term for inflammation of the mucous membranes of the bronchial tubes is
    a. pneumonia
    b. pneumonomycosis
    c. bronchitis
    d. bronchostenosis
    e. bronchiectasis

Answer: c

13. Which of the following statements about the pleura is CORRECT?
    a. It is a muscle that separates the abdominal and thoracic cavities.
    b. It is a membrane contained in the lungs that allows exchange of oxygen and carbon dioxide.
    c. It is cartilaginous rings that give support to the larynx.
    d. It is one of the lobes of the right lung.
    e. It is a membrane that covers the lung.

Answer: e

14. The condition characterized by attacks of difficult breathing and wheezing caused by spasms of the bronchial tubes is
    a. pleurisy
    b. asthma
    c. pneumonia
    d. bronchorrhagia
    e. aerophagia

Answer: b

15. The medical term for a surgical puncture to remove fluid from the lung is
    a. pneumocentesis
    b. pneumectomy
    c. thoracocentesis
    d. thoracotomy
    e. bronchostenosis

Answer: a

16. The medical term for incision into a lobe of the lung is
    a. lobectomy
    b. pneumonectomy
    c. lobotomy
    d. pharyngotomy
    e. thoracotomy

Answer: c

17. Which of the following medical terms denotes normal breathing?
    a. eupnea
    b. dyspnea
    c. apnea
    d. orthopnea
    e. fascia

Answer: a

18. The medical term that means a small tumor on a pedicle is
    a. neoplasm
    b. polyp
    c. metastatic
    d. nodular
    e. meatus

Answer: b

19. The medical term for a tumor of the liver is
    a. myoma
    b. hepatoma
    c. carcinoma
    d. chondroma
    e. polyp

Answer: b

20. The medical term for swallowing air is
    a. aerophagia
    b. aerotherapy
    c. aerophobia
    d. aerohydrotherapy
    e. aeroscope

Answer: a

21. The term for inflammation of the vertebrae is
    a. osteoporosis
    b. spondylitis
    c. spina bifida
    d. ankylosis
    e. meningitis

Answer: b

22. A loss of feeling or sensation is
    a. apnea
    b. anesthesia
    c. aspiration
    d. aerophagia
    e. asthma

Answer: b

23. Suture of a muscle is
    a. myopathy
    b. myoma
    c. myodynia
    d. myoplasty
    e. myorrhaphy

Answer: e

24. Difficult or labored breathing is termed
    a. eupnea
    b. tachypnea
    c. apnea
    d. dyspnea
    e. bradypnea

Answer: d

25. An occupational disease caused by inhalation of black dust is called
    a. melanosis
    b. pneumonosis
    c. silicosis
    d. siderosis
    e. pneumonomelanosis

Answer: e

26. The presence of pus in the pleural cavity is
    a. empyema
    b. pyosis
    c. pyemia
    d. pyothoracosis
    e. empyosis

Answer: a

27. Which of the following is a genetic disorder?
    a. atelectasis
    b. cystic fibrosis
    c. pertussis
    d. epiglottitis
    e. emphysema

Answer: b

28. An infectious disease that produces tubercles in the lungs is
    a. emphysema
    b. asthma
    c. pneumonia
    d. tuberculosis
    e. bronchitis

Answer: d

29. A whistling or sighing sound resulting from narrowing of the lumen of a respiratory passageway that is noted by use of a stethoscope is called
    a. stridor
    b. rhonci
    c. wheezes
    d. rales
    e. croup

Answer: c

30. A contagious respiratory infection characterized by onset of fever, chills, headache, and muscle pain is
    a. epiglottitis
    b. asthma
    c. atelectasis
    d. epistaxis
    e. influenza

Answer: e

UNIT 7   ENDOCRINE AND NERVOUS SYSTEMS

STUDENT OUTCOMES

Upon completion of this unit, you will be able to:

♦ Explain the main functions of the endocrine and nervous systems.

♦ Identify the organs and structures of the endocrine system.

♦ Identify the combining forms and suffixes related to the organs and structures of the endocrine system.

♦ Build and analyze medical terms related to the endocrine and nervous systems by completing the frames and reviews.

♦ Evaluate medical reports.

♦ Spell and pronounce medical terms by completing the audiocassette activities.

Unit 7: Endocrine and Nervous Systems

Multiple choice: Select the best answer.

1. The hormone PTH is produced by which of the following glands?
    a. parathyroid
    b. pituitary
    c. pancreas
    d. thymus
    e. thyroid

Answer: a

2. The adrenal glands are located superior to the
    a. liver
    b. kidneys
    c. pancreas
    d. gallbladder
    e. brain stem

Answer: b

3. How many parathyroid glands are present in the body?
    a. 2
    b. 3
    c. 4
    d. 5
    e. 6

Answer: c

4. The hormone that is responsible for uterine contractions during childbirth is
    a. glucagon
    b. FSH
    c. estrogen
    d. oxytocin
    e. progesterone

Answer: d

5. Giantism and dwarfism are both a result of improper functioning of hormones of which of the following glands
   a. pituitary
   b. adrenal
   c. thyroid
   d. pancreas
   e. thymus

Answer: a

6. The gland that regulates the body's metabolism is the
   a. pituitary
   b. pancreas
   c. adrenal
   d. thymus
   e. thyroid

Answer: e

7. Which of the following hormones helps control the calcium level in the blood?
   a. oxytocin
   b. insulin
   c. epinephrine
   d. FSH
   e. PTH

Answer: e

8. Which of the following hormones is responsible for the body being able to react to dangerous situations with increased responsiveness and energy?
   a. epinephrine
   b. insulin
   c. glucagon
   d. oxytocin
   e. ADH

Answer: a

9. The gland that produces the hormone responsible for maintaining secondary sex characteristics is the
   a. adrenal gland
   b. thyroid gland
   c. thymus gland
   d. pituitary gland
   e. pancreas

Answer: a

10. What is the function of the hormone glucagon?
    a. It lowers blood glucose levels.
    b. It increases blood glucose levels.
    c. It regulates the amount of salt in the body.
    d. It stimulates absorption of calcium.
    e. It regulates metabolism of the body.

Answer: b

11. The primary source of energy for living organisms is
    a. fat
    b. glucose
    c. salt
    d. water
    e. vitamin C

Answer: b

12. Symptoms of diabetes include all of the following EXCEPT
    a. polyuria
    b. polydipsia
    c. polyphagia
    d. anorexia
    e. hyperglycemia

Answer: d

13. When the membranes that cover the brain protrude or herniate through the opening of the skull, the condition is called
    a. cerebrosclerosis
    b. an encephaloma
    c. a meningocele
    d. a stroke
    e. a neuroglia

Answer: c

14. The inability to speak is called
    a. apnea
    b. aphasia
    c. anorexia
    d. dysphasia
    e. diplopia

Answer: b

15. The front lobe of the pituitary gland is called the
    a. anterior lobe
    b. posterior lobe
    c. inferior lobe
    d. superior lobe
    e. posterosuperior lobe

Answer: a

16. An orchidopexy is a surgical fixation of the
    a. ovaries
    b. adrenal gland
    c. pancreas
    d. testes
    e. liver

Answer: d

17. An endocrinologist treats patients who suffer from
    a. cerebral palsy
    b. a CVA
    c. meningitis
    d. myeloma
    e. diabetes

Answer: e

18. Which of the following glands is located on the front and sides of the trachea just below the larynx?
    a. thymus
    b. pituitary
    c. adrenal
    d. pancreas
    e. thyroid

Answer: e

19. The suprarenal glands are superior to the kidneys. This means that they are located
    a. above the kidneys
    b. below the kidneys
    c. in front of the kidneys
    d. behind the kidneys
    e. beside the kidneys

Answer: a

20. The inner part of the adrenal gland is called the
    a. cortex
    b. hypophysis
    c. medulla
    d. isthmus
    e. islets

Answer: c

21. Incision of the thyroid gland is termed
    a. thyrostomy
    b. thyrotomy
    c. thyropathy
    d. thyromegaly
    e. thyroidectomy

Answer: b

22. The abnormal condition of a pancreatic stone is
    a. pancreatitis
    b. pancreatopathy
    c. pancreatomegaly
    d. pancreatoma
    e. pancreatolithiasis

Answer: e

23. A disease characterized by polyuria, polydipsia, and polyphagia is
    a. diabetes mellitus
    b. myelomalacia
    c. hypercalcemia
    d. acromegaly
    e. jaundice

Answer: a

24. Another term for stroke is
    a. paraplegia
    b. cerebral palsy
    c. Parkinsonian syndrome
    d. cerebrovascular accident
    e. myelomalacia

Answer: d

25. A yellowish discoloration of the skin and eyes is
    a. metastasis
    b. acromegaly
    c. jaundice
    d. deglutition
    e. glycogenesis

Answer: c

26. Graves' disease is also known as
    a. hypothyroidism
    b. thyrotoxicosis
    c. myxedema
    d. cretinism
    e. thyrotropin

Answer: b

27. An enlargement of the thyroid gland is called a(n)
    a. adenoma
    b. neoplasm
    c. thyrotoxicosis
    d. goiter
    e. hyperplasia

Answer: d

28. Which condition is associated with hypothyroidism?
    a. Cushing's disease
    b. Parkinson's disease
    c. myxedema
    d. giantism
    e. hirsutism

Answer: c

29. A congenital defect characterized by incomplete closure of the spinal canal is
    a. shingles
    b. sciatica
    c. spondylosis
    d. hydrocephalus
    e. spina bifida

Answer: e

30. Choose the one diagnostic term that is NOT related to the others
    a. cerebrovascular accident
    b. trigeminal neuralgia
    c. stroke
    d. CVA
    e. apoplexy

Answer: b

UNIT 8   MUSCULOSKELETAL SYSTEM

STUDENT OUTCOMES

Upon completion of this unit, you will be able to:

♦ Explain the main functions of the musculoskeletal system systems.

♦ Locate and identify the major bones of the body.

♦ Explain the function of the vertebral column, and list the five main groups of bones in the vertebral column.

♦ Describe the function of joints.

♦ Identify the combining forms and suffixes related to the musculoskeletal system.

♦ Build and analyze medical terms related to the musculoskeletal system by completing the frames and reviews.

♦ Evaluate medical reports.

♦ Spell and pronounce medical terms by completing the audiocassette activities.

Unit 8: Musculoskeletal System

Multiple choice: Select the best answer.

1. The medical term for the suture of a bone is
   a. osteomalacia
   b. osteorrhaphy
   c. osteogenesis
   d. osteoarthritis
   e. osteosclerosis

Answer: b

2. The medical term that means the opposite of osteosclerosis is
   a. osteogenesis
   b. osteorrhaphy
   c. osteomalacia
   d. osteoarthritis
   e. none of the above is the opposite

Answer: c

3. The term for the shaft of a long bone is
   a. myeloblast
   b. epiphysis
   c. osteocyte
   d. periosteum
   e. diaphysis

Answer: e

4. A person with inflammation of a joint experiences
   a. costalgia
   b. cephalalgia
   c. arthrodynia
   d. chondritis
   e. osteodynia

Answer: c

5. Trauma to a joint that causes injury to the surrounding ligament is
    a. a strain
    b. a sprain
    c. torticollis
    d. tendinitis
    e. talipes

Answer: b

6. Encephalopathy is the medical term for a disease of the
    a. head
    b. covering of the brain
    c. brain
    d. skull
    e. spinal column

Answer: c

7. Intercostal muscles are located between the
    a. vertebrae and ribs
    b. fingers
    c. toes
    d. ribs
    e. vertebrae

Answer: d

8. Which type of fracture results when the broken ends of the bones are forced into one another?
    a. compound
    b. greenstick
    c. impacted
    d. simple
    e. open

Answer: c

9. Which of the following words is in its plural form?
   a. bursae
   b. vertebra
   c. phalange
   d. pleura
   e. all are in their plural forms

Answer: a

10. The term spondylitis means inflammation of the
    a. synovial fluid
    b. ribs
    c. fingers
    d. cartilage
    e. vertebrae

Answer: e

11. Intervertebral disks are composed of
    a. bone
    b. cartilage
    c. muscle fibers
    d. synovial fluid
    e. ligaments

Answer: b

12. The atlas supports the skull and is the
    a. first cervical vertebra
    b. first thoracic vertebra
    c. first lumbar vertebra
    d. sacrum
    e. coccyx

Answer: a

13. The ribs articulate with the
    a. cervical vertebrae
    b. thoracic vertebrae
    c. lumbar vertebrae
    d. sacrum
    e. coccyx

Answer: b

14. A patient with lumbodynia is experiencing pain in the
    a. knee
    b. ankle
    c. head
    d. back
    e. chest

Answer: d

15. The tail of the vertebral column is termed the
    a. carpal
    b. calcaneum
    c. coccyx
    d. sacrum
    e. lamina

Answer: c

16. The term myotomy means incision into
    a. the bone marrow
    b. the cartilage
    c. a tendon
    d. the spinal cord
    e. a muscle

Answer: e

17. The function of a tendon is to
    a. attach bone to bone
    b. attach muscle to bone
    c. attach muscle to muscle
    d. attach cartilage to bone
    e. attach vertebra to vertebra

Answer: b

18. An individual with quadriplegia has paralysis of
    a. one upper extremity
    b. both upper extremities
    c. one lower extremity
    d. both lower extremities
    e. all extremities

Answer: e

19. The Achilles tendon is located in the
    a. back
    b. upper arm
    c. foot
    d. knee
    e. chest

Answer: c

20. The term cervicofacial refers to the face and
    a. head
    b. neck
    c. chest
    d. hand
    e. brain

Answer: b

21. A disease in children in which an inefficient mineralization of the bone-forming tissue causes deformities is
    a. osteochondroma
    b. rickets
    c. myelomalacia
    d. meningocele
    e. chondritis

Answer: b

22. A directional word meaning near the point of attachment to the trunk is
    a. lateral
    b. distal
    c. proximal
    d. superior
    e. inferior

Answer: c

23. A physician who specializes in the use of x-rays for diagnosis and treatment of disease is a
    a. radiography
    b. radiologist
    c. physiologist
    d. roentgenologist
    e. b and d

Answer: e

24. The membrane that lines the brain and spinal cord is the
    a. epithalamus
    b. vertebral
    c. lamina
    d. meninges
    e. gray matter

Answer: d

25. An excessive amount of calcium in the blood is termed
    a. calicosis
    b. hypercalcemia
    c. calcitonin
    d. hypocalcemia
    e. calciuria

Answer: b

26. A lateral curvature of the spine is called
    a. lordosis
    b. sciatica
    c. necrosis
    d. scoliosis
    e. kyphosis

Answer: d

27. Another name for osteitis deformans is
    a. osteoporosis
    b. Paget's disease
    c. polio
    d. Pott's disease
    e. osteomyelitis

Answer: b

28. A neuromuscular disorder characterized by severe muscular weakness and progressive fatigue is
    a. muscular dystrophy
    b. talipes
    c. sequestrum
    d. myasthenia gravis
    e. torticollis

Answer: a

29. The second vertebra is identified as
    a. T2
    b. L2
    c. S2
    d. C2
    e. V2

Answer: d

30. A disease characterized by excessive uric acid is
    a. rheumatoid arthritis
    b. crepitation
    c. contracture
    d. gout
    e. acidosis

Answer: d

UNIT 9   CARDIOVASCULAR SYSTEM

STUDENT OUTCOMES

Upon completion of this unit, you will be able to:

♦ Explain the main function of the cardiovascular and lymphatic systems.

♦ Identify the hearts three distinct layers.

♦ Name the four chambers of the heart, and state the function of each chamber.

♦ Identify the combining forms and suffixes related to the cardiovascular and lymphatic systems.

♦ Explain the conduction pathway of the heart.

♦ Analyze an electrocardiogram strip during systole and diastole.

♦ Build and analyze medical terms related to the cardiovascular and lymphatic systems by completing the frames and reviews.

♦ Evaluate medical histories.

♦ Spell and pronounce medical terms by completing the audiocassette activities.

Unit 9: Cardiovascular and Lymphatic Systems

Multiple choice: Select the best answer.

1. Oxygenated blood leaves the heart through which of the following vessels
   a. pulmonary vein
   b. superior vena cava
   c. inferior vena cava
   d. pulmonary artery
   e. aorta

Answer: e

2. Which of the following is inferior to the mitral valve?
   a. right atrium
   b. right ventricle
   c. left atrium
   d. left ventricle
   e. pulmonary vein

Answer: d

3. The medical term for suturing a vein is
   a. phleborrhaphy
   b. venosclerosis
   c. phlebostenosis
   d. venotomy
   e. phleborrhexis

Answer: a

4. The term aortostenosis denotes that there is a(n)
   a. rupture of the aorta
   b. softening of the aorta
   c. narrowing of the aorta
   d. expansion of the aorta
   e. disease of the aorta

Answer: c

5. Which of the following conditions can be detected on an electrocardiogram?
   a. tachycardia
   b. bradyphagia
   c. phlebostenosis
   d. aneurysm
   e. hemangioma

Answer: a

6. When a weakness in a vessel causes the ballooning of the wall of the vessel, the condition is called a(n)
   a. thrombolysis
   b. angioma
   c. arteriolith
   d. aneurysm
   e. arteriopathy

Answer: d

7. Each of the following abbreviations is matched with the correct corresponding term EXCEPT
   a. IVC—inferior ventricular contractions
   b. CHF—congestive heart failure
   c. LV—left ventricle
   d. MI—myocardial infarction
   e. SA—sinoatrial

Answer: a

8. The cervical lymph nodes are located in the
   a. armpit
   b. neck
   c. groin
   d. abdomen
   e. chest

Answer: b

9. Streptococcal infection that causes damage to the heart valves and heart muscle is
    a. Raynaud's syndrome
    b. an embolus
    c. varicose veins
    d. rheumatic heart disease
    e. transient ischemic attack

Answer: d

10. The tricuspid valve is located between which two chambers of the heart?
    a. right atrium and left atrium
    b. right atrium and right ventricle
    c. right atrium and left ventricle
    d. right ventricle and left ventricle
    e. left atrium and left ventricle

Answer: b

11. Which of the following is the medical term for rupture of a vein?
    a. phleborrhexis
    b. phleborrhaphy
    c. phlebostenosis
    d. venotomy
    e. venosclerosis

Answer: a

12. The interventricular septum separates the left ventricle from the
    a. right atrium
    b. left atrium
    c. right ventricle
    d. myocardium
    e. pericardium

Answer: c

13. How many flaps are present in the bicuspid valve?
    a. 1
    b. 2
    c. 3
    d. 4
    e. 5

Answer: b

14. The superior vena cava receives blood from the
    a. right atrium
    b. legs and torso
    c. pulmonary artery
    d. head and arms
    e. right ventricle

Answer: d

15. The membranous sac that encloses the heart is the
    a. myocardium
    b. pericardium
    c. septum
    d. endocardium
    e. epicardium

Answer: b

16. The minute air sacs of the lungs that contain millions of capillaries are
    a. pulmonary veins
    b. valves
    c. pulmonary capillaries
    d. alveoli
    e. pulmonary arteries

Answer: d

17. Which of the following medical terms is singular?
    a. septum
    b. atria
    c. cardia
    d. bacteria
    e. all are singular

Answer: a

18. The SA node is located in the
    a. aortic arch
    b. right ventricle
    c. left atrium
    d. left ventricle
    e. right atrium

Answer: e

19. After the electrical impulse of the heart passes through the AV node, it travels next to the
    a. SA node
    b. bundle of HIS
    c. Purkinje fibers
    d. bundle branches
    e. mitral valve

Answer: b

20. The term for the external muscular layer of the heart is the
    a. myocardium
    b. endocardium
    c. pericardium
    d. epicardium
    e. atrium

Answer: d

21. The chamber of the heart that receives oxygen-poor blood from all tissues EXCEPT the lungs is the
    a. right atrium
    b. left atrium
    c. right ventricle
    d. left ventricle
    e. all are correct

Answer: a

22. A disease characterized by an abnormal hardening of the arteries is called
    a. cardiomegaly
    b. aortomalacia
    c. arteriosclerosis
    d. aortopathy
    e. arteriospasm

Answer: c

23. The relaxation phase of the heart is
    a. systole
    b. diastole
    c. tachycardia
    d. bradycardia
    e. angiectasis

Answer: b

24. The medical term for a tumor composed of lymph vessels is a(n)
    a. lymphoma
    b. angioma
    c. myoma
    d. hematoma
    e. lymphangioma

Answer: e

25. Major lymph node sites include all of the following EXCEPT
    a. pectoral nodes
    b. cervical nodes
    c. axillary nodes
    d. inguinal nodes
    e. armpit nodes

Answer: a

26. A condition in which the heart is unable to pump adequate amounts
    of blood to tissues and organs is
    a. arteriosclerosis
    b. rheumatic heart disease
    c. congestive heart failure
    d. hypertension
    e. aortic coarctation

Answer: c

27. Blood vessel obstruction caused by a traveling mass of undissolved matter is
    a. a thrombus
    b. a patent ductus arteriosus
    c. a fibrillation
    d. an arrhythmia
    e. an embolus

Answer: e

28. A soft-blowing sound caused by turbulent blood flow is a
    a. rale
    b. gallop
    c. bruit
    d. wheeze
    e. crackle

Answer: c

29. Medication used to dissolve a thrombus is an
    a. antiemetic
    b. anticoagulant
    c. antihistamine
    d. antiarrhythmic
    e. antigen

Answer: b

30. Temporary blood supply interference to the brain without permanent brain damage
    is called a (an)
    a. EBV
    b. MVP
    c. MI
    d. TIA
    e. HIV

Answer: d

UNIT 10   SPECIAL SENSES: THE EYES AND EARS

STUDENT OUTCOMES

Upon completion of this unit, you will be able to:

♦ List and briefly describe each of the special senses of the body.

♦ Identify the major structures and functions of the eye.

♦ Identify the major structures and functions of the ear.

♦ Identify the combining forms and suffixes related to the organs and structures of the special senses.

♦ Build and analyze medical terms related to the eyes and ears by completing the frames and reviews.

♦ Evaluate medical reports.

♦ Spell and pronounce medical terms by completing the audiocassette activities.

Unit 10: Special Senses

Multiple choice: Select the best answer.

1. An excision of a part or all of the eyelid is called a(n)
   a. blepharectomy
   b. ophthalmectomy
   c. blepharotomy
   d. keratorrhexis
   e. keratotomy

Answer: a

2. The part of the eye that is composed of nerve endings and is responsible for the reception and transmission of light impulses is the
   a. sclera
   b. choroid
   c. iris
   d. retina
   e. cornea

Answer: d

3. Which of the following is the medical term for far-sightedness?
   a. diplopia
   b. hyperopia
   c. myopia
   d. erythropia
   e. xanthopia

Answer: b

4. The colored muscular layer that surrounds the pupil is the
   a. sclera
   b. retina
   c. iris
   d. choroid
   e. cornea

Answer: c

5. Which of the following is the name of the ducts that collect and drain tears?
   a. auricle
   b. incus
   c. malleus
   d. choroid
   e. lacrimal

Answer: e

6. A person with dacryadenalgia has pain in
   a. the middle ear
   b. a tear gland
   c. the eardrum
   d. the retina
   e. the eyelid

Answer: b

7. The part of the eye that is transparent and allows the entrance of light to the interior of the eye is the
   a. choroid
   b. pupil
   c. sclera
   d. cornea
   e. iris

Answer: d

8. Which of the following is a part of the external ear?
   a. malleus
   b. stapes
   c. auricle
   d. eustachian tube
   e. cochlea

Answer: c

9. The structure that leads from the middle ear to the nasopharynx is the
   a. tympanic membrane
   b. eustachian tube
   c. malleus
   d. cochlea
   e. auricle

Answer: b

10. The structure of the inner ear that helps an individual maintain equilibrium is the
    a. cochlea
    b. stapes
    c. incus
    d. semicircular canal
    e. tympanic membrane

Answer: d

11. A visual examination of the eustachian tube is called a(n)
    a. ophthalmoscopy
    b. salpingoscopy
    c. otoscopy
    d. ophthalmoscope
    e. salpingoscope

Answer: b

12. The white of the eye is also known as the
    a. sclera
    b. retina
    c. choroid
    d. cornea
    e. iris

Answer: a

13. Plastic surgery of the ear is called
    a. blepharoplasty
    b. keratotomy
    c. otoscopy
    d. salpingoscopy
    e. otoplasty

Answer: e

14. The term labyrinth is sometimes used when referring to the
    a. choroid
    b. inner ear
    c. external ear
    d. middle ear
    e. eustachian tube

Answer: b

15. Which of the following medical terms is a synonym for ophthalmodynia?
    a. ophthalmalgia
    b. ophthalmectomy
    c. ophthalmoplegia
    d. ophthalmoscopy
    e. none of the above

Answer: a

16. The medical term otalgia means
    a. softening of the ear
    b. rupture of the ear drum
    c. suture of the ear
    d. difficult hearing
    e. pain in the ear

Answer: e

17. Which of the following medical terms relates to vision?
    a. blepharoptosis
    b. ophthalmalgia
    c. otodynia
    d. diplopia
    e. dacryorrhea

Answer: d

18. Each of the following is a structure of the ear EXCEPT
    a. cochlea
    b. incus
    c. choroid
    d. malleus
    e. stapes

Answer: c

19. ENT is the abbreviation for
    a. eyes, nose, and throat
    b. eyes, nose, and tympanic membrane
    c. ears, nose, and tympanic membrane
    d. ears, nose, and throat
    e. eyelids, nose, and throat

Answer: d

20. A physician who specializes in treatment of eye disorders is a(n)
    a. optometrist
    b. ophthalmologist
    c. physiologist
    d. psychologist
    e. neurologist

Answer: b

21. A narrowing or stricture of the eustachian tube is called
    a. salpingectomy
    b. salpingosis
    c. salpingostenosis
    d. salpingotomy
    e. salpingoplasty

Answer: c

22. An involuntary contraction or twitching of the eyelid is
    a. choroiditis
    b. choroidopathy
    c. blepharoplasty
    d. blepharitis
    e. blepharospasm

Answer: e

23. The structure that provides the blood supply for the entire eye is the
    a. choroid
    b. sclera
    c. cornea
    d. retina
    e. iris

Answer: a

24. Rupture of the cornea is called
    a. choroidorrhexis
    b. choroiditis
    c. keratitis
    d. keratorrhexis
    e. tympanorrhexis

Answer: d

25. The synonym for double vision is
    a. myopia
    b. hyperopia
    c. diplopia
    d. nearsightedness
    e. farsightedness

Answer: c

26. Excessive intraocular pressure, often leading to blindness, is
    a. astigmatism
    b. glaucoma
    c. esotropia
    d. cataract
    e. amblyopia

Answer: b

27. The technical term for complete color blindness is
    a. chromatophilia
    b. chromatophobia
    c. achromia
    d. achromatopsia
    e. chromatopsia

Answer: d

28. Impaired hearing that is part of the aging process is
    a. prebycusis
    b. tinnitus
    c. vertigo
    d. paracusis
    e. anacusis

Answer: a

29. An inflammation of the middle ear is called
    a. labyrinthitis
    b. tympanitis
    c. mastoiditis
    d. otitis media
    e. conjunctivitis

Answer: d

30. A synonym for sty is
    a. hordeolum
    b. variola
    c. vertigo
    d. cerumen
    e. choroiditis

Answer: a

ANSWER KEY TO TABLE FRAMES IN UNIT 7, ENDOCRINE SYSTEM

Frame 7-5 Refer to Table 7-1 to complete Frames 7-5 and 7-6.

Define the term hormone(s).
Hormones are chemical substances produced by specialized cells of the body.

Frame 7-6 List two common characteristics of hormones.
1. **Hormones are released slowly in minute amounts directly into the bloodstream.**
2. **Hormones are produced primarily by endocrine glands.**
3. **Most hormones are inactivated or excreted by the liver and kidneys.**

Frame 7-21 Refer to Table 7-2 to complete Frames 7-21 through 7-26. The two hormones produced by the neur/o/hypophysis are **antidiuretic hormone (ADH) and oxytocin.**

Frame 7-22 Define the following abbreviaions:
GH **growth hormone**
TSH **thyroid-stimulating hormone**
ADH **antidiuretic hormone**

Frame 7-23 Briefly state two functions of the ADH.
ADH decreases volume of urine excreted and increases volume of water reabsorbed in the kidney.

Frame 7-24 Briefly state two functions of GH.
GH stimulates bone and body growth

Frame 7-25 The hormone that causes contraction of the uterus during childbirth is **oxytocin.**

Frame 7-26 Write the abbreviation of the hormone that initiates sperm production in men. **FSH** follicle-stimulating hormone

Frame 7-38 Refer to Table 7-3 to complete Frames 7-38 through 7-40. The thyroid gland produces two hormones that regulate the body's metabolism (rate at which food is converted into heat and energy). These hormones are called **thyroxine and triiodothyronine.**

Frame 7-39 Calcium and phosphate levels in the blood are controlled by the hormone **calcitonin.**

Frame 7-40 The three hormones produced by the thyroid gland are **thyroxine, triiodothyronine, and calcitonin.**

Frame 7-53 Refer to Table 7-4 to complete this frame. The major function of PTH is to regulate levels of **calcium and phospHate.**

Frame 7-60 Refer to Tables 7-5 and 7-6 to complete Frames 7-60 through 7-65. The three hormones produced by the adrenal cortex are **aldosterone, cortisol, and androgens.**

Frame 7-61 Identify the hormone produced by the adrenal cortex that maintains secondary sex characeristics. **Androgens** regulate the amount of salts in the body: **aldosterone.**

Frame 7-62 Two hormones produced by the adrenal medulla are epinephrine, also called **adrenaline.**

Frame 7-63 epinephrine (or adrenaline) helps the body to cope with dangerous situations. Nerves transmit the message of fear to the glands, which react by rushing adrenaline to all parts of the system. Epinephrine is also called **adrenaline.**

Frame 7-64 When a person is experiencing a stressful situation, the adrenal medulla produces adrenaline, also called **epinephrine.**

Frame 7-65 The hormone produced by the adrenal medulla that raises blood pressure is called **norepinephrine** or **noradrenaline.**

Frame 7-69 Refer to Table 7-7 to complete frames 7-69 through 7-71. The two hormones produced by the pancreas are **insulin and glucagon.**

Frame 7-70 Determine the pancreat/ic hormone that does the following:

lowers blood sugar: **insulin**
increases blood sugar: **glucagon**

Frame 7-71 How does insulin lower blood sugar?
Insulin lowers blood sugar by promoting the movement of glucose to the body cells.

SUPPLEMENTAL INSTRUCTIONAL ACTIVITIES

Medical Reports

Medical reports related to various medical specialties provide supplementary instructional activities so students can continue to learn and apply the medical language as it is used in the health-care industry.

A dictionary exercise and an evaluation of each medical report provides experiences that help students to learn numerous practical applications of medical terminology.

The medical reports can be used for group activities, oral reports, or individual assignments. All of the reports are designed to reinforce and expand the terminology covered in the textbook.

Unit 2 Digestive System

The following reports are related to the medical specialty called gastroenterology.

Medical Report 2–1: GI Evaluation

Dictionary Exercise

Underline the following terms in this report. Use a medical dictionary and Appendix E, "Abbreviations," to write a definition of each word or abbreviation. This exercise helps you to master the terminology in this report.

adhesions_____

anicteric_____

appendectomy_____

bruits_____

carotids_____

CVA_____

cholecystectomy_____

cholecystitis_____

cholelithiasis_____

cyanosis_____

defecate_____

duodenal_____

edema_____

epigastric_____

etiology_____

flatus_____

ganglion_____

GI_____

heme_____

hepato_____

hydronephrosis_____

lymphadenopathy_____

nephrolithiasis_____

splenomegaly_____

stool_____

syndrome_____

thyromegaly_____

tonsillectomy_____

ulcer_____

ultrasound_____

Medical Report 2–1: GI Evaluation

Read the medical report out loud.

<u>HISTORY OF PRESENT ILLNESS</u>: Patient is a 35-year-old white woman who is here because of right-sided abdominal pain of 4 months' duration. The patient's abdominal pain dates back 2 years ago when she first had intermittent sharp epigastric pain. Each episode lasted 2 to 4 hours. Eventually she was diagnosed as having cholecystitis with cholelithiasis and underwent cholecystectomy. Three to five large calcified stones were found. I am not certain if small stones were also present.

Her postoperative course was uneventful until 4 months ago when she began having continuous deep right-sided pain. This pain took a crescendo pattern and peaked several weeks ago when family stress was also at its climax. Since then the pain has taken a decrescendo pattern, and the patient acknowledges that it is pretty much back down to the baseline achy sensation. It does not cause any nausea or vomit. It does not trigger any urge to defecate, nor is it alleviated by passage of flatus.

<u>PAST MEDICAL HISTORY</u>: Significant only for tonsillectomy, appendectomy, and cholecystectomy. She also had a ganglion of the hand removed.

<u>PHYSICAL EXAMINATION</u>: Markedly obese. Wt 235 lb. BP 96/66. P 76. Normocephalic, atraumatic. PERRLA, EOMs intact. Anicteric. Normal oral cavities. Neck: no lymphadenopathy or thyromegaly. Carotids: normal without bruits. No CVA tenderness. Abdomen: obese, normal bowel sounds, soft diffuse tenderness on deep palpation without localized tenderness in the right upper quadrant area. There was no hepato or splenomegaly. Rectal: normal sphincter tone, heme-negative stool. Extremities: no cyanosis, clubbing, or edema.

Recent laboratory studies revealed a normal CBC and normal chemistry with a bilirubin of 0.5, AST of 14, ALK of 11, GGT of 16, and alkaline phosphatase of 83. Abdominal ultrasound revealed no biliary dilation. The pancreas was well visualized and normal. Kidneys showed no evidence of hydronephrosis. An upper GI was also performed recently and revealed no abnormalities.

<u>IMPRESSION</u>: Intermittent low-grade right-sided abdominal pain, etiology unclear. One possible differential diagnosis includes retained common bile duct stones, which are highly unlikely considering the quality of the pain and the completely normal liver function test. Duodenal ulcer is always a possibility, although again the characteristics of the pain are not

typical. Hepatic flexure syndrome is one of the most common causes of pain in this area. Adhesions with pain of the right upper quadrant as a result of cholecystectomy also needs to be considered. Lastly, an occult nephrolithiasis needs to be considered in spite of the normal ultrasound of the kidney.

Evaluation of Medical Report 2–1: GI Evaluation

1. Refer to Figure 2–1, Digestive System (textbook), to determine where the gallbladder is located in relation to the liver?

2. Examine Figure 2–5, Accessory Organs of Digestion (textbook). What duct does the doctor suspect might have retained stones?

3. Was her preoperative pain constant?

4. How does her most recent postoperative episode of discomfort (pain) differ from the initial pain she described?

5. Has she had any other surgeries of the GI system?

6. If so, what were they? If not, which systems were involved?

7. Were the laboratory findings within normal limits?

8. There is the possibility of an ulcer. Refer to Figure 2–1, Digestive System (textbook), to determine which part of the bowel is involved? Is this the most common site?

9. What x-ray showed no abnormalities?

10. Which structures are examined in an upper GI? Refer to Appendix C, "Radiographic Procedures," barium swallow.

Medical Report 2-2: Operative Report—Left Colon Resection

Dictionary Exercise

Underline the following terms in this report. Use a medical dictionary and Appendix E, "Abbreviations," to write a definition of each word or abbreviation. This exercise helps you to master the terminology in this report.

anastomosis_____

annular_____

carcinoma_____

cavity_____

cm_____

colocolostomy_____

dissection_____

distal_____

endotracheal_____

flexure_____

gastrocolic_____

greater curvature_____

hepatic_____

lavage_____

ligated_____

lumen_____

metastases_____

midline_____

operative_____

peritoneal_____

proximal_____

resection_____

splenic_____

subcutaneous_____

supine_____

tenia_____

umbilicus_____

vital signs_____

Medical Report 2–2: Operative Report—Left Colon Resection

Read the Medical report out loud.

PREOPERATIVE DIAGNOSIS: Annular lesion of distal transverse colon proximal to splenic flexure, consistent with carcinoma.

POSTOPERATIVE DIAGNOSIS: Same, without evidence of peritoneal implantation or hepatic metastases.

OPERATION: Left colon resection including takedown of splenic flexure with end-to-end transverse descending colocolostomy.

<u>FINDINGS AND PROCEDURE</u>: The patient was placed supine on an operating table, and a general endotracheal anesthetic was administered uneventfully by Dr. Rosen. The abdomen was prepared with Hibiclens and alcohol. The operative field was draped with sterile towels and sheets.

A primary upper midline incision was used extending to the left around the umbilicus. Initial exploration of the peritoneal cavity was essentially unremarkable, except for an annular constricting lesion in the distal transverse colon. There were no other significant intra-abdominal findings.

The operation was commenced by placing a wound protector drape and an upper-hand and a balfour retractor. The peritoneal attachments in the lateral gutter were freed with direct inspection of the splenic attachments, which were freed by electric knife dissection without further event. Gradually the entire splenic flexure was released, and a site high on the greater curvature of the stomach where the gastrocolic omentum is located was serially clamped, divided, and ligated with 2-0 Dexon.

A section of transverse colon 6 cm from the lesion was identified and freed of surrounding fat and vessels. The mesentery could then be lifted up and inspected directly. The left colic vessels were clamped, divided, and ligated doubly with 2-0 Dexon. Additional vessels supplying the tumor and the section to be removed were serially clamped, divided, and ligated with 2-0 Dexon. The distal specimen was freed of surrounding fat and vessels, and the specimen was removed proximally and distally using GI stapling devices.

A transverse colocolostomy was fashioned along the tenia after the specimen had been resected using a GI stapling device to perform the anastomosis and after closure of the defect with running 3-0 GI Dexon in the mucosa and interrupted 3-0 silk in the muscular serosa. A very satisfactory lumen, under no tension and with good blood supply, appeared to be accomplished by these maneuvers.

Fresh gloves and instruments were used to complete the procedure. The operative area was lavaged with physiologic saline, and returns were clear. The intestinal contents were replaced. The wound protector drape was removed. The abdomen was closed in layers with O Dexon and metallic staples in the skin.

As closure was accomplished, 50,000 U Bacitracin and 100 cc of saline lavage were used in the subcutaneous tissues. Sponge, needle, and instrument counts were correct. Blood loss was minimal. Operating time was 2 hours. The procedure was uneventful. The patient's vital signs remained stable throughout, and he was transferred to the recovery room in satisfactory condition.

Evaluation of Medical Report 2–2: Operative Report—Left Colon Resection

1. Refer to Figure 2–1, Digestive System (textbook), to identify the location of the lesion.

2. Describe the shape of the lesion.

3. Was the lesion benign or malignant?

4. Did the lesion spread to the liver?

5. The doctor did a colocolostomy. What is the difference between that and a colostomy?

6. Is the greater curvature on the lateral or the medial side of the stomach?
7. What is an anastomosis?

8. What are vital signs?

Medical Report 2–3: Colonoscopy and Polypectomy

Dictionary Exercise

Underline the following terms in this report. Use a medical dictionary and Appendix E, "Abbreviations," to write a definition of each word or abbreviation. This exercise helps you to master the terminology in this report.

cecum_____
colonoscope_____
colonoscopy_____
digital_____
distal_____
diverticular_____
endoscope_____
fiberoptic_____
flexure_____
hepatic_____
ileum_____
junction_____
mm_____
paternal_____
polypectomy_____
polyps_____
rectosigmoid_____

sessile_____

snared_____

terminal_____

Medical Report 2–3: Colonoscopy and Polypectomy

Read the Medical report out loud.

<u>PREOPERATIVE DIAGNOSIS</u>: Family history of colon cancer and polyps.

<u>POSTOPERATIVE DIAGNOSIS</u>: Sessile polyp of the distal rectum. Small sessile polyp at the rectosigmoid junction. Small sessile polyp of the hepatic flexure. Probable diverticular disease of the transverse colon.

<u>OPERATION</u>: Colonoscopy and polypectomy.

<u>INDICATIONS</u>: This 60-year-old gentleman has a strong history of colon polyps and malignancy. Two paternal uncles had colon cancer, both are deceased from this disease. Father had colonoscopy for removal of polyps. This patient comes in now for colonoscopy and cancer and polyp surveillance.

After digital examination of the anal canal and rectum, the Olympus fiberoptic CF 20L colonoscope was rotated into the sigmoid colon from the rectum. At the rectosigmoid junction a 4- to 5-mm sessile polyp was identified. The endoscope was advanced first to the splenic flexure and then into a well-haustrated transverse colon. First, the hepatic flexure was reached, and then the instrument was advanced down into the cecum. The cecal landmarks were well identified, and the terminal ileum was entered.

At this point the endoscope was slowly withdrawn. At the hepatic flexure there appeared to be a small, flat polyp on one of the haustral folds. This was snared, lifted up, removed, and retrieved. It appeared that there were one or two diverticular openings in the transverse colon. There was no associated inflammation.

The endoscope was further removed, and at 16 cm there was a well-defined semipedunculated polyp. This was removed using the self-opening Wilson-Cooke electrocautery snare and a No. 3 coagulation current setting on the Valley Laboratory Electrosurgical Unit. This polyp was also retrieved with suction. An additional smaller lesion was seen just at the rectosigmoid junction at 14 cm, and another in the distal rectum. All were removed and retrieved in similar fashion. There was no evidence of bleeding.

The patient tolerated the procedure exceedingly well. In view of his family history and the multiplicity of polyps, he should have follow-up colonoscopy in 1 year.

Evaluation of Medical Report 2–3: Colonoscopy and Polypectomy

1. What is the difference between a sessile polyp and a pedunculated polyp?

2. How many sessile polyps did the patient have?

3. Was the endoscope advanced into the small bowel? If so, which part of the small bowel?

4. As the endoscope was being removed, a well-defined semipedunculated polyp was identified. How far into the bowel was it located?

5. What is a diverticulum?

6. This patient had one or two diverticular openings. In which part of the large bowel were they identified?

7. Why did the doctor recommend an annual colonoscopy?

Unit 3 Urinary System

The following medical reports are related to the medical specialties called nephrology and urology.

Medical Report 3–1: Nephrology Consultation

Dictionary Exercise

Underline the following terms in this report. Use a medical dictionary and Appendix E, "Abbreviations," to write a definition of each word or abbreviation. This exercise helps you to master the terminology in this report.

ascites_____
BUN_____
Ca_____
CBC_____
chronic_____
CO_2_____
creatinine_____
dysphagia_____
Hct_____
Hgb_____
hydration_____
hypovolemia_____
IVP_____
K_____
lethargy_____
malaise_____
Mg_____
mmHg_____
Na_____
peripheral_____
pyelonephritis_____
renal_____
scan_____
SGOT_____
SGPT_____
turgor_____
hypochondrium_____
WBC_____

Medical Report 3-1: Nephrology Consultation

Read the Medical report out loud.

HISTORY OF PRESENT ILLNESS: This 57-year-old white man was admitted to the hospital yesterday with a history of progressive lethargy, weakness, dysphagia, constipation, and generalized malaise. These symptoms have been present for the last 3 to 4 days.

During his last hospitalization on January 18,19xx, preoperative investigation revealed a BUN 32 and a creatinine of 2.8, and there was no documentation of any BUN or creatinine at the time of discharge. He had a normal IVP.

It was noticed that he had a urinary tract infection with *E. coli* at that time, and hence he was discharged with Bactrim.

PHYSICAL EXAMINATION: Revealed a 57-year-old man, a little lethargic, well oriented. His BP was 136/74 mmHg. Tongue pink and a little dry. Neck: carotid pulsations normal. Skin: decreased in turgor at present. Heart sounds normal. No gallop. Lungs with normal breath sounds. Abdomen is full with operative scar in the right hypochondrium, with ascites present. Extremities: no peripheral edema. Well perfused. Peripheral pulsations normal.

LABORATORY: Blood chemistry on 08/20/xx: Na 134. K 4.7. CO_2 80. Cl 100. BUN 128. Creatinine 10.0. Random blood sugar 117. Blood chemistry on 10/13/xx: Na 139. K 4.4. CO_2 18. Cl 107. BUN 138. Creatinine 7.6. Fasting blood sugar 110. Ca 8.3. P 5.5. Uric acid 19.7. Total protein 5.8 Albumin 2.4. Mg 3.4. Alkaline phosphatase 41.2. SGPT 59. SGOT 62. CBC: WBC 6.2 with Hgb 13.3; Hct 38.4; platelets 246,000. Urinalysis has shown specific gravity of 1.012. No protein or hemoglobin; WBC 2-3; RBC 0-1; bacterial cells 1+.

IMPRESSION: The patient has chronic renal failure of several years' duration with compromised renal function. His postoperative course was uneventful except for complaint of slight reduction of urinary output. There has been no documentation of renal function at the time of discharge. The patient was given Bactrim, following which the patient developed symptoms of uremia, and on investigation, the patient's renal function has markedly deteriorated in the course of 5 days. It is my presumption that the patient's chronic renal failure, which was in a delicate balance, has further deteriorated with Bactrim. The Bactrim has been discontinued for 24 hours now. There has been improvement in the creatinine level, from 10 to 7.6 mg%. His BUN is still high, and it appears the patient is still in hypovolemia and needs further hydration.

In addition, the patient has pyelonephritis of several years' duration, and analysis of the urine yesterday does not reveal any evidence of persistence of the infection. The patient might also have renal functional impairment secondary to chronic pyelonephritis.

Review of the record and the patient: reveals no evidence of acute ischemic renal failure. His serum magnesium is high, and the patient has received some Milk of Magnesia at home.

If the patient does not show any further improvement in the next 24 hours, suggest obtaining a renal scan with blood flow studies.

Evaluation of Medical Report 3-1: Nephrology Consultation

1. Were the results of the preoperative BUN and creatinine studies abnormal?

2. Which organ function is evaluated with those laboratory tests?

3. What is an IVP?

4. Why has his skin turgor decreased?

5. Has the patient experienced any decrease in urinary output?

6. Where is the right hypochondriac region?

7. What is ascites?

8. Did the patient have any swelling of the extremities?

9. What part of the kidney has inflammation?

Medical Report 3-2: Probable Urosepsis

Dictionary Exercise

Underline the following terms in this report. Use a medical dictionary and Appendix E, "Abbreviations," to write a definition of each word or abbreviation. This exercise helps you to master the terminology in this report.

appendectomy_____
dehydration_____
embolism_____
esterase_____
hysterectomy_____
nitrates_____
organomegaly_____
pulmonary_____
sp. gr._____

urosepsis_____
UTI_____

Medical Report 3–2: Probable Urosepsis

Read the medical report out loud.

HISTORY OF PRESENT ILLNESS: The patient is an 81-year-old white woman who is admitted through the emergency department (ED) at Stanford Hospital with dehydration, urinary tract infection (UTI), and vaginitis. She was totally uncooperative at the time that I saw her, so the history is pieced together from the ED report and past medical records.

PAST MEDICAL HISTORY AND SURGERIES: The patient had a fractured leg in 1978. She had a left hip prosthesis. She had a hysterectomy and appendectomy. She was in Marshall Hospital in 1985 with blood clots in the leg and possible pulmonary embolism. She has had consequent problems with easy bleeding. MEDICATIONS: Presently she is taking Ampicillin for a urinary tract infection, and the drug apparently did not work. This was prescribed on August 24. At that time a Foley catheter was also placed. The patient presented to the ED today being clinically worsened. She was noted at that time to have a UTI and also a purulent vaginal drainage.

PHYSICAL EXAMINATION: Vital Signs: T 96°F. P 80. B/P 104/60. HEENT: severely limited because the patient would not open her eyes or mouth. No lesions were seen. Chest: clear, although I was not able to listen to all lung fields. Breasts: unremarkable. Heart: regular. Abdomen: soft. No organomegaly or masses. No tenderness noted. Rectal/vaginal: not completed because of lack of patient compliance. Extremities: The patient had multiple skin tears and bruises on her extremities.

LABORATORY DATA: The patient had a white count of 12.1. The renal panel was unremarkable. Sodium was slightly down at 135. The urinalysis was significant for positive nitrates, positive leukocyte esterase, and an sp. gr. of 1.025.

ASSESSMENT:
1. Urinary tract infection, probably urosepsis
2. Dehydration
3. Vaginitis

PLAN: Blood cultures, urine cultures and vaginal cultures were done. The patient was started on IV antibiotics. Will also administer IV fluids and treat presumptively with Terazol cream at this time.

Evaluation of Medical Report 3–2: Probable Urosepsis

1. Do you suppose the vaginitis is a complication from taking Ampicillin? Check with a *Physician's Desk Reference* for side effects of this drug.

2. Did the vaginal discharge consist of pus?

3. What caused her pulmonary embolism?

4. Did she have any enlargements of the abdominal organs?

5. How was she hydrated?

6. Was her white count significant?

7. Was the specific gravity within normal limits?

Medical Report 3–3: Ureteral Calculus

Dictionary Exercise

Underline the following terms in this report. Use a medical dictionary and Appendix E, "Abbreviations," to write a definition of each word and abbreviation. This exercise helps you to master the terminology in this report.

bilateral_____
calculus_____
cm_____
cystoscope_____
cystoscopy_____
cytology_____
extubate_____
genitalia_____
lithotomy_____
orifices_____
panendoscope_____
proximal_____
radiolucent_____
renal pelvis_____
retrograde pyelogram_____
stent._____
strictured_____
ureter_____

ureteral_____

ureteroscope_____

urethra_____

Medical Report 3–3: Ureteral Calculus

Read the Medical report out loud.

PREOPERATIVE DIAGNOSIS: Obstruction, right proximal ureter.

POSTOPERATIVE DIAGNOSIS: Right proximal ureteral calculus.

PROCEDURE: Cystoscopy, bilateral retrograde pyelograms, right rigid and flexible ureteroscopy, and insertion of right double J stent.

The patient was taken to the cystoscopy suite, and general anesthesia was induced and maintained in the usual fashion without difficulty. The patient was then placed in the lithotomy position, and the external genitalia were prepared and draped in the usual sterile fashion. A No. 23 French ACMI panendoscope was inserted into the patient's urethra blindly and into the bladder. A urine specimen was collected for cytology. The urethra was tight to this size scope, but it does fit. Inspection of the bladder with both straight- and right-angle lenses showed no abnormalities of the bladder. The ureteral orifices were located in the usual position. The prostate was inspected with a straight lens and was also felt to be normal. It was minimally obstructive. The urethra was also normal. Bilateral retrograde pyelograms were taken with a bulb-tip catheter. These clearly showed a foreign body in the proximal right ureter. This is a radiolucent object. A guidewire was obtained and passed up the right ureter beyond the stone and into the renal pelvis without difficulty. A dilating catheter was obtained, and the distal ureter was dilated without difficulty for 10 minutes using the Olbert dilating catheter. Once this is done, the cystoscope was removed and a ureteroscope was obtained and passed into the ureter without difficulty. However, just above the true pelvis, the ureter was very strictured. Stricture of the ureter was dilated with a balloon catheter, and then another stricture was encountered. A second balloon catheter was used to dilate this stricture, and a third stricture was encountered. It was apparent that the middle portion of the ureter has numerous strictures and narrow areas, and it was impossible to pass the rigid scope beyond this point. Then a flexible No. 7 French scope was obtained and was passed through a cystoscope and over a guidewire up the ureter until the stone was encountered. It would not go beyond the stone. With active flushing using a syringe, the stone could be seen at the end of the flexible ureteroscope, confirming the diagnosis of right ureteral calculus. However, nothing could be used to manipulate the stone, and the flexible ureteroscope was removed. The ureter was further dilated with rigid dilators. However, the larger of these would not go up the ureter, and I did not force them. Then the rigid ureteroscope was obtained and passed back into the ureter, and again I encountered numerous strictures of the mid ureter and was

unable to pass the scope to the level of the stone. Ureteroscopy was then abandoned. A No. 7

French 26-cm double J stent was passed over the guidewire in the ureter without difficulty using a cystoscope. A good loop formed in the kidney as well as in the bladder. The bladder was then drained. The procedure was now completed. The patient was awakened, extubated, and taken to the recovery room in good condition.

Evaluation of Medical Report 3–3: Ureteral Calculus

1. What caused the ureteral obstruction?

2. What is a cystoscope?

3. What is the difference between a retrograde pyelogram and an IVP?

4. Why was the urologist unable to remove the ureteral calculus?

5. Which part of the ureter was obstructed?

6. What is a stent?

7. How many scopes did the doctor use? Name them.

8. Did the radiolucent object appear white or dark on the x-ray?

Unit 4 Integumentary System

The following medical reports are related to the medical specialty called dermatology. Plastic surgeons also do procedures to enhance this system.

Medical Report 4-1: Redundant Facial and Neck Skin with Submental Adipose Tissue

Dictionary Exercise

Underline the following terms in this report. Use a medical dictionary and Appendix E, "Abbreviations." to write a definition of each word and abbreviation. This exercise helps you to master the terminology in this report.

adipose_____
auricular_____
cannula_____
cc_____
cm_____
defatted_____
electrocautery_____
fold_____
hemostasis_____
nasolabial_____
occipital_____
platysma_____
posterior_____
redundant_____
rhytidectomy_____
skin flaps_____
subcutaneous_____
subcuticular_____
submental_____
temporal_____
tragus_____
undermined_____

Medical Report 4–1: Redundant Facial and Neck Skin with Submental Adipose Tissue

Read the Medical report out loud.

OPERATION: Rhytidectomy with submental SAL and triangle hair-sparing temporal incision.

PROCEDURE: With the patient in the supine position, the hair was trimmed appropriately and shaved. The hair also was tied in rubber bands. A standard C-shaped incision was made in the temporal area, coming down in front of the ear and going in behind the tragus. The incision then went up the back of the ear and curved in a wavy fashion back into the occipital hair-bearing skin. After marking the incisions, both sides were then injected with approximately 20 cc of Webster's solution, including the submental area all the way across. The incisions were then made, and the skin and subcutaneous tissue were undermined out to the nasolabial fold area and down into the neck. Bleeding was controlled with electrocautery.

Because of the looseness in the SMAS and platysmal muscle, the parotid fascia was then incised and undermined enough to allow the SMAS to be brought back behind the ear, and this was tacked in place with interrupted 5-0 white twisted nylon sutures. Some of the SMAS was also incised and sewed to the edge of the posterior SMAS. This tightened the platysma and SMAS tissue. Once again, the bleeding was controlled with electrocautery.

A 0.5-cm incision was then made in the submental crease, and through this as well as the side access through the posterior incisions, the submental adipose tissue was suctioned using a small suction cannula. This gave a honeycombed effect that greatly softened the submental area and helped to recreate a bit of an angle, which was not present before, in the cervical mandibular area.

The submental incision was then closed with interrupted 5-0 Vicryl sutures. After hemostasis was again maintained with electrocautery, the skin was redraped and the excess removed. Closure was carried out with interrupted 4-0 nylon sutures and staples within the hair-bearing areas. Where there was only hair on one side, half-mattress sutures were used. In front of the ear, 5-0 Vicryl subcuticular sutures were used, and the skin over the tragus was carefully defatted before closure using a running 6-0 nylon suture. Also, in order to gain a little bit more lift in the jowl area without raising the hairline, a small triangle of skin about 15 cm long and 2 cm wide was removed underneath the temporal hairline. The posterior auricular area was closed with a running 5-0 nylon suture, and the area between the ear and the hair-bearing area was closed to the subcuticular area with interrupted 5-0 Vicryl sutures.

At the end of the procedure, the air and residual blood were rolled out from underneath the skin flaps. There was very little bleeding during the procedure, and hemostasis appeared to be well maintained. The skin color was very good, and the patient was dressed with Xeroform gauze over the suture lines in front of and behind the ears, fluffs, and Kerlix rolls, which were also carried underneath the chin. The patient was then transferred to the recovery area in satisfactory condition.

Evaluation of Medical Report 4-1: Redundant Facial and Neck Skin with Submental Adipose Tissue.

1. Did they make an incision under the chin?

2. What method did they use to control bleeding?

3. Where is the tragus located?

4. What suture did they use to close behind the ear?

Medical Report 4-2: Burn, Right Hand

Dictionary Exercise

Underline the following terms in this report. Use a medical dictionary and Appendix E, "Abbreviations." to write a definition of each word and abbreviation. This exercise helps you to master the terminology in this report.

ulnar_____
palmar_____
prophylaxis_____
nodal_____
cm_____
eschar_____
anesthesia_____
topical_____
systemic_____

Medical Report 4–2: Burn, Right Hand

Read the medical report out loud.

<u>PRESENT ILLNESS</u>: The patient is a 36-year-old woman referred by Dr. Hernandez for treatment of a burn involving her right hand. The injury occurred at 6:30 this morning as a result of a spark from a hair dryer. This involved the ulnar palmar aspect of her right hand. She was seen by Dr. Hernandez today, who provided tetanus prophylaxis. She has been on doxycycline for treatment of an ongoing nodal infection.

<u>PHYSICAL EXAMINATION</u>: A 2 cm by 1.5 cm area of pale eschar is present over the ulnar palmar aspect of the right hand. There is anesthesia over the eschar. The intrinsic muscles demonstrate normal function. She also has normal tenderness function. There is no loss of range of motion or pain with motion.

<u>IMPRESSION</u>: I advised the patient that this likely represents a full-thickness skin burn. She demonstrates no signs of deeper injury, such as to the muscles, tendons, or bones at this time. We will observe the area. This will be treated with Silvadene on a topical basis. I do not think that she requires systemic antibiotics, although she is currently on doxycycline.

Evaluation of Medical Report 4–2: Burn, Right Hand

1. Does the patient have feeling in her hand in the burn area?

2. Is it the back or the palm of the hand that received the burn?

3. Was it her thumb side that was burned?

4. Did the doctor prescribe oral antibiotics?

5. Did she lose any muscle function?

Medical Report 4-3: Lesion of Left Ring Finger

Dictionary Exercise

Underline the following terms in this report. Use a medical dictionary and Appendix E, "Abbreviations," to write a definition of each word and abbreviation. This exercise helps you to master the terminology in this report.

biopsy_____

block_____

cryotherapy_____

dermatologist_____

digital_____

ellipsoid_____

excision_____

inflammation_____

neurovascular_____

subdermal_____

transverse_____

Medical Report 4–3: Lesion of Left Ring Finger

OPERATION: Excision of lesion of left ring finger and complex repair of defect.

ANESTHESIA: Local through digital block.

FINDINGS: The patient is a 32-year-old man referred by his dermatologist for treatment of a recurrent lesion of his left ring finger. The patient states that the process began approximately 6 months ago with a rapidly enlarging lesion that became tender. It was treated initially with cryotherapy and antibiotics, which resulted in a gradual recurrence. This was foillowed by shave biopsy, which resulted in a rapid recurrence and enlargement. The risks, benefits, and alternatives to a definitive excisional biopsy were therefore discussed with the patient, who consented to the procedure.

PROCEDURE: The patient was first placed on a course of preoperative antibiotics to treat local inflammation and possible local infection. On the day of the procedure he was taken to the operating room and placed on the operating table in the supine position. The entire left hand and arm were prepped and draped in the usual manner. Adequate anesthesia was achieved through a digital block by depositing approximately 2 cc of 2% lidocaine near the neurovascular bundles. The lesion was identified and marked within a transverse ellipsoid for an excision. The specimen was excised at the subdermal level with the scalpel. The wound was then irrigated, and hemostasis was restored with electrocautery. Care was taken to identify any residual diseased tissue. The proximal skin flap was then elevated to allow approximation and repair. A dissection was performed over a distance of greater than 1 cm. This allowed advancement of this flap and approximation with minimal tension. The flap was held in position with sutures of 5-0 Vicryl. The wound was then dressed with Xeroform gauze and soft cotton sponges. The finger was immobilized in an aluminum splint secured with tube gauze.

Evaluation of Medical Report 4–3: Lesion of Left Ring Finger

1. What did the doctor do to the lesion?

2. How long did the patient have the lesion?

3. How did the dermatologist treat the lesion initially?

4. Where did the doctor administer the anesthetic block?

5. How deep did the surgeon cut to remove the lesion?

Unit 5 Reproductive System

The following medical reports are related to the medical specialties called gynecology, for female reproductive diseases/disorders, and urology, for male reproductive diseases/disorders.

Female Reproductive System

Medical Report 5-1: Carcinoma, Lower Inner Breast, Clinical Stage 1, Discovered by Mammography

Dictionary Exercise

Underline the following terms in this report. Use a medical dictionary and Appendix E, "Abbreviations," to write a definition of each word and abbreviation. This exercise helps you to master the terminology in this report.

arcus senilis_____

asymptomatic_____

axillary_____

biopsy_____

carcinoma_____

chronologic_____

cm_____

estrogens_____

everted_____

hallux valgus_____

inframammary_____

mammography_____

mastectomy_____

menarche_____

menopause_____

metastatic_____

mucoid_____

nodule_____

non-palpable_____

OU_____

pendulous_____

quadrant_____

retroverted_____

sequelae_____

subcutaneous_____

supraclavicular_____

symmetrical_____

thelarche_____

varicosity_____

Medical Report 5–1: Carcinoma, Lower Inner Breast, Clinical Stage 1, Discovered by Mammography

Read the medical report out loud.

When first seen, this 82-year-old divorced woman was asymptomatic with respect to breast disease but, on routine mammography, was found to have a 1.3-cm nodule in the lower inner right breast, quite near the inframammary line. It had some characteristics of malignancy, and a breast biopsy was recommended. The lesion was definitely non-palpable by the patient, myself, and Dr. Pargett, and when the breast biopsy was done on January 15, 19xx, it was truly a very soft, mucoid lesion, diagnosed as a mucinous carcinoma (so-called colloid carcinoma) of about 10 mm in diameter without vascular invasion. The tumor was also estrogen- and progesterone-positive. The Kl proliferating cell antibody, K167, was low, and the diploidy analysis revealed a near-diploid lesion. She subsequently has had a complete blood count, chemistry panel, chest x-ray, and bone scan, which showed no obvious metastatic disease. She wished to consider radiation therapy, and she was referred to Dr. Franklin Huberty for this treatment, but after full discussion, she decided against proceeding. She opted instead for modified radical mastectomy, the definitive treatment for this type of carcinoma. The nature of this surgery, pre- and post-operative care, and possible complications such as swelling of the upper extremity on the same side, wound problems, infection, bleeding, pulmonary and vascular complications were explained on several occasions at great length, and I believe she understands. Also, she has donated a unit of her own blood to be used as a component in a fibrin glue application during the procedure, in an effort to prevent postoperative residual axillary and subcutaneous flap fluid collection.

Thelarche occurred about age 12, with menarche at age 11. The patient was always very generously developed and was at least a D cup throughout life. She had her first of four children at age 32 and the last at age 42, nursing only the first; she was told there was not enough milk in spite of the size of her breasts. Menopause occurred when she was in her early 50s. She was placed on estrogens, which were gradually reduced, and she stopped them about 20 years ago. The patient takes a minimum of caffeine beverages. She does not use a hair dye. Review of systems and past medical history is unremarkable except for fractures of both wrists without sequelae. Family history is significant as follows: Father, died at age 54 with colon cancer, mother at age 96 of "old age." The sister, aged 77, had breast cancer but apparently has remained free of disease. She also had a stroke. The other sister, at age 80, is still living. She had uterine cancer.

Physical examination reveals a well-developed, well-nourished, and attractive woman who appears much younger than her chronologic age. Vital signs are within normal limits. She has arcus senilis, OU, and wears glasses for reading and driving. Breasts: generous and symmetrical, as well as pendulous. There is a recent right lower inner quadrant scar. No other masses. The nipples are everted. No axillary or supraclavicular findings. Pelvic exam reveals a retroverted uterus. Spine and extremities: There is hallux valgus bilaterally, and one small venous varicosity of the right lateral knee. No edema, no stasis changes.

Evaluation of Medical Report 5–1: Carcinoma, Lower Inner Breast, Clinical Stage 1, Discovered by Mammography

1. Did this patient have symptoms which caused her to seek medical attention?

2. Was the nodule located above or below the breast?

3. Could the doctors feel the nodule?

4. Did they treat the nodule with x-ray therapy?

5. At what age did she start her menses?

6. At what age did her breast develop?

7. What is wrong with her eyes?

8. Are her nipples of normal contour?

9. Why did they have her donate a unit of her own blood prior to surgery?

10. In what direction is her uterus flexed?

11. What is wrong with her feet?

Medical Report 5–2: Bilateral Hypomastia

Dictionary Exercise

Underline the following terms in this report. Use a medical dictionary and Appendix E, "Abbreviations," to write a definition of each word and abbreviation. This exercise helps you to master the terminology in this report.

antibiotic_____

augmentation_____

bilateral_____

bovie_____

cc_____

dermis_____

electrocautery _____

hemostasis_____

hypomastia_____

inferior_____

inframmary_____

intercostal_____

irrigated_____

lumen_____

mammoplasty _____

periareolar_____

perioperative_____

scalpel_____

subcuticular_____

submuscular_____

subpectoral_____

titrated_____

Medical Report 5–2: Bilateral Hypomastia

Read the medical report out loud.

OPERATION: Bilateral submuscular augmentation mammoplasty.

ANESTHESIA: Regional by intercostal nerve blocks supplemented with local infiltration and intravenous sedation.

FINDINGS: The patient is a 26-year-old woman who is dissatisfied with the volume of her breasts. Following a discussion of the risks, benefits, and alternatives to breast augmentation, the patient has consented to the operation. We have planned to place submuscular prostheses through periareolar incisions.

PROCEDURE: The patient was first treated in the preoperative holding area where 1 g of Keflin was provided as a perioperative antibiotic. The margins of the breast, including the inframammary fold, were marked with a standard gential violet pen. Intravenous sedation was titrated to tolerance. She was then taken to the operating room and placed on the operating table in a supine position. The anterior thorax was prepped and draped from bedline to bedline in the usual manner. Intercostal nerve blocks were performed by bilaterally depositing 1 cc of ¼% Marcaine beneath ribs two through six. This was supplemented by the direct infiltration into the operative field of ½% lidocaine with epinephrine.

Bilateral inferior periareolar incisions were marked, then performed with the scalpel. The dissection was continued through the breast tissue with the bovie to the level of the pectoralis fascia. The fascia and the underlying muscle were divided in the direction of the fibers to enter the subpectoral plane. The submuscular pocket was enlarged to accommodate the implant. The limits of the dissection medially were the sternum, superiorly the second rib, laterally the mid-anterior line, and inferiorly the inframammary fold. In creating the pocket, it extended laterally beneath the serratus anterior muscles and inferiorly beneath the anterior rectus fascia to obtain maximal submuscular coverage of the prosthesis. Identical pockets were created on each side and checked for symmetry. The pockets were then thoroughly irrigated with a saline solution, and meticulous hemostasis was obtained through pinpoint electrocautery. Multiple implants were then obtained and placed into the pockets as "sizers." Optimal contour consistent with her preoperative volume desires was achieved with implants of 200 cc. Two McGhan style 200-cc double-lumen implants were then obtained. The outer lumens were evacuated of all air, and no saline was added. The pockets were again thoroughly irrigated with the saline solution as well as an antibiotic solution. The implants were placed into the pockets. The repair was performed in layers. The pectoralis muscle was repaired with interrupted sutures of 3-0 Vicryl. The breast tissue was approximated with interrupted sutures of 3-0 Vicryl. The subcutaneous tissue and deep dermis of the skin were repaired with inverting sutures of 4-0 Vicryl. Final skin approximation was with a running subcuticular suture of 4-0 Prolene. The wounds were further reinforced with Steri-strips.

1. Evaluation of Medical Report 5–2: Bilateral Hypomastia

2. What was wrong with her breasts?

3. What is an augmentation mammoplasty?

4. Where was the incision made?

5. Were individual sutures closing the skin used?

Medical Report 5–3: Breast Reduction

Dictionary Exercise

Underline the following terms in this report. Use a medical dictionary and Appendix E, "Abbreviations." to write a definition of each word and abbreviation. This exercise helps you to master the terminology in this report.

AB_____
abdominoplasty_____
adenopathy_____
areolae_____
cholecystitis_____
cm_____
everted_____
gastric_____
gravida_____
inferiorly_____
inframammary_____
intertriginous_____
mammoplasty _____
morbid_____
obesity_____
panniculus_____
para_____
paraesthesias_____
pendulous_____
ptotic_____
reduction_____
retractions_____
stapling_____
striae_____
transverse_____

Medical Report 5–3: Breast Reduction

Read the medical report out loud.

<u>PRESENT ILLNESS</u>: The patient is a 37-year-old woman who presents for consideration of a reduction mammoplasty as well as a possible abdominoplasty.

The patient is 5 feet 5 inches tall and currently weighs 125 lb. At one time her weight was 255 lb; however, she was treated by gastric stapling. Her current weight has been stable for some

time. Her current bra size is stable at 36DD. Her maximal size was a 46EEE.
The patient has no history of breast lumps, biopsies, or other breast surgery. There is no
family history of breast cancer, although there is a family history of large breasts. This
involves her mother and her two daughters. Her youngest daughter wears a 34B bra at
age 11.

The patient is a gravida II, para II, AB 0, who breastfed her second daughter for 1 year. At
that time she was a 46 "huge."

The patient's symptoms include pain of the neck and back of 10 years' duration. She also has
grooving from her shoulder straps as well as paraesthesias of the fingers. She has been tested
and may have carpal tunnel syndrome. She also has a history of intertriginous rashes.

The patient's abdominal problem is the presence of a large abdominal panniculus following the
massive weight loss after the gastric stapling. Gastric stapling was performed in December of
1986 and repeated in February of 1988.

PAST HISTORY: Hypertension. History of morbid obesity. History of cholecystitis.
Gastric stapling in Reno, Neveda, in December of 1986. She also had a simultaneous hiatal
hernia repair. The gastric stapling was repeated in February of 1988. She also had a TVH-
BSO in April of 1987. She had a cholecystectomy in September of 1988.

PHYSICAL EXAMINATION: The breasts are large and pendulous, with numerous striae
present superiorly. The nipples are located at 30 cm from the sternal notch on the right and 32
cm on the left. This is 6 cm below the inframammary fold on the right and 6.5 cm on the left.
Numerous striae are present in the superior hemispheres of the breast. The transverse
diameter of the areolae are 5.5 cm on the right and 6.0 cm on the left. No masses are palpable
on either breast, and there is no axillary or supraclavicular adenopathy. There are no skin
retractions and the nipples are everted. There is decreased sensation to the nipples.

The abdomen is significant for a large superior hockey-stick incision. This is due to a left
subcostal incision, which crosses midline, and a right subcostal incision, which meets the left
subcostal incision. The umbilicus is displaced inferiorly approximately 1 cm. There is a 2-cm
apron present. Beneath this is a Pfannenstiel incision. The skin is severely ptotic and lacking
in elasticity and compliance.

IMPRESSION: I advised the patient that she is a candidate for the reduction mammoplasty, as
well as the abdominoplasty. In particular, the reduction mammoplasty should be covered
through her insurance policy.

Risks, benefits, and alternatives to the reduction mammoplasty as well as the abdominoplasty
were discussed with the patient in detail. Risks discussed in regards to the reduction included

pain, hemorrhage, infection, reaction to medications, unfavorable scarring, breast asymmetry, loss of nipple-areolar sensation or possible total loss of the complexes, loss of the breast, chronic drainage of the breast, asymmetry, unnatural contours to the breast, unnatural position of the nipples, and need for secondary or revisional surgery. The patient understands this and has consented to the operation.

Evaluation of Medical Report 5–3: Breast Reduction

1. How many pregnancies have been successful for this patient?

2. What makes this person a good candidate for a reduction mammoplasty?

3. Is mammary hypertrophy a familial trait?

4. What symptoms does this patient have involving her fingers due to mammary hypertrophy?

5. Where is her rash?

6. What is this client's abdominal problem?

7. Does her skin have good turgor?

Male Reproductive System

Medical Report 5-4: Impotence and Penile Prosthesis

Dictionary Exercise

Underline the following terms in this report. Use a medical dictionary and Appendix E, "Abbreviations," to write a definition of each word and abbreviation. This exercise helps you to master the terminology in this report.

afebrile_____
benign_____
hormonal_____
hypertension_____
impotence_____
manipulation_____
mg_____

penile_____

prn_____

prosthesis_____

qid_____

Medical Report 5–4: Impotence and Penile Prosthesis

Read the medical report out loud.

PRESENT ILLNESS: The patient is a 55-year-old white man with a long-standing history of hypertension, which was controlled initially with propranolol and subsequently with Lopressor two tablets per day. The patient, however, has suffered with problems of impotence, and despite hormonal manipulation, he has had no improvement of his impotence. The patient is admitted at this time for an elective placement of a penile prosthesis.

HOSPITAL COURSE: On the day following admission the patient was taken to the operating room, where he underwent placement of a Flexirod penile prosthesis. The patient's postoperative course was benign. He was ambulating with no pain, was afebrile, and had prompt healing of his incision. He was discharged on his third postoperative day with Keflex 250 mg qid and Tylenol No. 3 prn and was to be followed up in the urology outpatient clinic in 1 week. Discharge instructions regarding activity and diet were given.

Evaluation of Medical Report 5–4: Impotence and Penile Prosthesis

1. What was the main reason the patient sought medical help?

2. What medical treatment was given prior to surgery?

3. What type of prosthesis did the urologist use?

4. Did the patient have postoperative problems?

5. Did the patient have difficulty walking postoperatively?

6. How many times a day did the patient take the antibiotic?

Medical Report 5–5: Arterial and Venous Leak Impotence

Dictionary Exercise

Underline the following terms in this report. Use a medical dictionary and Appendix E, "Abbreviations," to write a definition of each word and abbreviation. This exercise helps you to master the terminology in this report.

afebrile_____

angiodynography_____

arterial_____

bulbocavernosus_____

cremasteric_____

dribble_____

erection_____

external_____

genitalia_____

girth_____

impotence_____

libido_____

normotensive_____

nocturia_____

patellar_____

peripheral_____

plantar_____

pulses_____

terminal_____

tid_____

varicosities_____

venous_____

Medical Report 5–5: Arterial and Venous Leak Impotence

I saw Omar Khan, a 68-year-old gentleman, who for the past 6 months or so has noted decreased ability to achieve full erection. The girth is not as good, and on penetration, he tends to lose his erection very quickly. He does take a long time to achieve orgasm, and as I have pointed out to him, this is a normal part of the aging process. His libido has also dropped quite dramatically. He has no voiding symptoms at all, other than some mild terminal dribble and occasional nocturia.

His current medications include Coumadin, atenolol, and Lanoxin. He has a very detailed impotence history filled out for me.

The major thrust of this appointment was because of this diminished libido and diminished girth. Apparently there is a lot of satisfaction within their relationship even without intercourse.

On examination he was afebrile and normotensive. The abdomen examined benignly. He had normal external genitalia. Rectal examination revealed a 10-g benign prostate. His peripheral pulses were present and equal. He did have varicosities in both lower legs. Neurological examination revealed normal patellar, ankle, and plantar responses; normal bulbocavernosus, anal, and cremasteric reflexes; and normal vibration sensation.

His fasting glucose, testosterone, LH, prolactin, and FSH levels were all within normal limits.

By description, I believe he probably has a combination of arterial and venous leak impotence. His diminution in libido may be a protective mechanism.

I have started him on Yocon in increasing increments, to build up to 2 tid to help his libido and perhaps increase blood flow. He is to call me and let me know how this works for him.
In the interim I am going to get angiodynography to assess his vascular status.

Evaluation of Medical Report 5–5: Arterial and Venous Leak Impotence

1. What does this gentleman's doctor feel is the source of his problem?

2. Which part of the extremities demonstrate varicose veins?

3. Does this patient have a decrease in penile sensation and reflexes?

4. How often does the client have to take Yokon?

What will the angiodynography prove?

Unit 6 Respiratory System

The following medical reports are from a specialty within internal medicine called pulmonary specialist for lung diseases/disorders.

Medical Report 6–1: Pulmonary Function Report (Pre- vs Post-comparison)

Dictionary Exercise

Underline the following terms in this report. Use a medical dictionary and Appendix E, "Abbreviations," to write a definition of each word and abbreviation. This exercise helps you to master the terminology in this report.

bronchodilators_____
expiratory_____
function_____
inhalation_____
normoxemia_____
pulmonary_____
SOB_____
vital capacity_____

Medical Report 6–1: Pulmonary Function Report (Pre- vs Post-comparison)

Read the medical report out loud.

SMOKING HISTORY: 90 pack-years.

DIAGNOSIS: SOB.

COMMENTS: Ratio analysis: ABG—PH 7.38, PCO_2 78, HCO_3 22, SAT 94%.

CALIBRATION: 3.00 L expected, 2.98 L measured.

INTERPRETATION: A mild decrease in forced vital capacity. A moderate decrease in forced expiratory volume in 1 second. The timed vital capacity is mildly reduced. Maximum midflow is severely decreased. There is no significant improvement in airflow following inhalation of the bronchodilators.

IMPRESSION: Mild limitation to the airflow. Arterial blood gas analysis on room air on this patient reveals normoxemia with normal acid-base status.

Evaluation of Medical Report 6-1: Pulmonary Function Report

1. Did this patient have any difficulty in breathing?

2. What was the presenting diagnosis?

3. What was the hydrogen ion concentration?

4. What was the level of bicarbonate radical?

5. What was the partial pressure of carbon dioxide? (Clue: This patient is retaining carbon dioxide.)

Medical Report 6-2: Left Empyema

Dictionary Exercise

Underline the following terms in this report. Use a medical dictionary and Appendix E, "Abbreviations," to write a definition of each word and abbreviation. This exercise helps you to master the terminology in this report.

afebrile_____
aspiration_____
atraumatic_____
Babinski's_____
bacillus_____
bilaterally_____
bronchoscopy_____
brushings_____
cachectic_____
carcinoma_____
CVA_____
cyanosis_____
diathesis_____
DTR_____
edema_____
edentulous_____
empyema_____
EOM_____
exudate_____
genitalia_____
granulomas_____

hematemesis_____

hemoptysis_____

laryngeal_____

neurological_____

normocephalic_____

orthopnea_____

PERRLA_____

pharynx_____

plantar_____

PND_____

pneumonectomy_____

presacral_____

purulent_____

rectal_____

squamous_____

staphylococcus_____

thoracostomy_____

thoracotomy_____

uncircumcised_____

wedge resection_____

Medical Report 6–2: Left Empyema

Read the medical report out loud.

CHIEF COMPLAINT: The patient is a 70-year-old man who is admitted with a left empyema.

PRESENT ILLNESS: This patient relates a history of actually not feeling well since his last lung surgery in February 19XX. He had a history of TB treated by wedge resection in the left upper and lower lobes in July 19XX. In February the patient was discovered to have a squamous cell carcinoma of the lung and underwent a left pneumonectomy. In December 19XX the patient had one episode of hemoptysis lasting approximately 4 days, when it resolved spontaneously.

On the morning of 05/20/9X, the patient had some blood-streaked sputum with persistent coughing and was seen in the emergency department. He was treated with tetracycline and was told to make an appointment in the surgery clinic.

The patient returned again on 05/21/9X with a history of hemoptysis, and at that time he was afebrile and denied any purulent sputum. The patient is a nonsmoker. All his cultures have always been negative for acid-fast bacillus. The patient denies any bleeding or diathesis.

The patient underwent bronchoscopy in May 19XX for episodes of hemoptysis. At that time brushings were taken, but there was no evidence of tumor or granulomas. There was no active bleeding at the time of bronchoscopy.

The patient was seen for follow-up every 3 months and began to notice the onset of a feverish feeling and lethargy. X-rays revealed a new air-filled level in the left thorax. Needle aspiration in the surgery clinic revealed purulent exudate with subsequent growth of staphylococcus.

The patient is admitted today for chest tube drainage and possible surgery of empyema of the left chest.

REVIEW OF SYSTEMS: The patient denies anymore hemoptysis, hematemesis; chest pain, shortness of breath, PND, orthopnea, or symptoms of claudication. The patient does state that during his previous surgery in 19XX, the nerve to his voice box was cut on one side.

PHYSICAL EXAMINATION: Reveals a somewhat cachectic, pleasant man in no acute distress. HEENT: atraumatic, normocephalic. PERRLA, EOMs intact. Mouth: edentulous. No exudates in the posterior pharynx. TMs are intact. Canals clear. Hearing is decreased bilaterally, secondary to artillery injury in WW II and Korea. Voice is high pitched and consistent with recurrent laryngeal nerve injury. Chest: There is a scar under the left breast from previous surgery with some retraction. There is decreased fremitus in the left chest. No breath sounds are present in the left chest. Transmitted breath sounds are present on the left from the right. Right lung fields are clear. Back: no CVA tenderness. No presacral edema. Abdomen: doughy with bowel sounds. Femoral pulses intact. Genitalia: both testes in the scrotum. Uncircumcised man. No hernia. Rectal: negative, good tone. Extremities: no clubbing, cyanosis, or edema. Neurological: physiologic. Rest of neurological examination is essentially unremarkable other than recurrent nerve injury in the left. Babinski's is plantar bilaterally. DTRs brisk.

PLAN: The patient will be brought into the hospital and placed on low-dose heparin, and a series of x-rays will be obtained. After radiologic visualization of the left thorax, tube thoracostomy drainage will be attempted to the left chest wall. If this is unsuccessful, the patient may need formal thoracotomy for drainage.

Evaluation of Medical Report 6–2: Left Empyema

1. How was this patient's tuberculosis treated?

2. What type of cancer did the patient have?

3. Did the patient have any postoperative complications?

4. What is the difference between sputum and saliva?

5. Why did the doctor do a needle aspiration?

6. What did the exudate look like?

7. Did the patient have any sudden shortness of breath at night?

8. Did he have to sleep in a "propped up" position?

9. When the doctor checked the neurological reflexes of his toes, did they point upward or downward?

10. If a tube cannot be inserted in the left chest, what can be done to remove the fluid?

Medical Report 6-3: Bronchogenic Carcinoma

Dictionary Exercise

Underline the following terms in this report. Use a medical dictionary and Appendix E, "Abbreviations," to write a definition of each word and abbreviation. This exercise helps you to master the terminology in this report.

asthma_____
biopsy_____
bronchial_____
bronchogenic_____
bronchoscopy_____
carcinoma_____
circumscribed_____
decortication_____
desensitized_____
dyspneic_____
hemopneumothorax_____
lesion_____
pneumothorax_____
preoperatively_____
pulmonary function test_____
thoracotomy_____
transfusions_____

Medical Report 6–3: Bronchogenic Carcinoma

This 52-year-old white widow developed a lesion in the left lung superior segment about a year and a half ago. She was studied at the county hospital, and bronchoscopy was done on several definite occasions and a needle biopsy last January. No definite diagnosis was made. She developed a pneumothorax following the needle biopsy and required closed tube drainage for about 10 days. Recent x-rays demonstrate the tumor as increasing in size. The patient has had bronchial asthma in 1983 while in Texas and was desensitized and placed on Bronchosol, Bronchotabs, and intermittent positive-pressure breathing. She is now on terbutaline 5 mg tid. She has smoked a ½ pack daily until about 2 years ago, when she quit. At the present time she feels perfectly well but does get dyspneic on exertion. She has gained weight to 140 lbs.

In 1972 she was hospitalized with a spontaneous hemopneumothorax and bled out into her right chest cavity, which required multiple transfusions and ultimately a right thoracotomy and decortication.

X-rays of the chest demonstrate a circumscribed tumor mass in the superior segment of the left lobe, which has almost doubled in size in the past year.

IMPRESSION: Bronchogenic carcinoma. The patient should have a left thoracotomy and resection of the left lower lobe. I would like to have a pulmonary function test performed preoperatively.

Evaluation of Medical Report 6–3: Bronchogenic carcinoma

1. What two diagnostic procedures were done at the county hospital?

2. What complication followed the needle biopsy?

3. What did they do correct the pneumothorax?

4. Why did they remove the visceral pleura from the right lung?

Medical Report 6–4: Pleural Atelectasis

Dictionary Exercise

Underline the following terms in this report. Use a medical dictionary and Appendix E, "Abbreviations," to write a definition of each word and abbreviation. This exercise helps you to master the terminology in this report.

adenopathy_____

arthritis_____

atelectasis_____

auscultation_____

bitemporal_____

bronchoscopy_____

bruits_____

carotids_____

cephalalgia_____

clubbing_____

cyanosis edema_____

endobronchial_____

ENT_____

fiberoptic_____

fundoscopic_____

gallop_____

hepato_____

lesion_____

myalgia_____

neurological_____

parasternal_____

percussion_____

PERRLA_____

PI_____

pleural_____

splenomegaly_____

sputum_____

URI_____

Medical Report No. 6–4: Pleural Atelectasis

CHIEF COMPLAINT: This 62-year-old housewife was referred for evaluation of cough and chest pain.

PRESENT ILLNESS: She states her present illness began with a URI over Thanksgiving, which was manifested by cephalalgia, bitemporal in nature; sore throat; myalgia; and cough. She was treated initially with cough syrup and antibiotics, and a chest x-ray was done, which showed right pleural atelectasis. This information was obtained per her telephone conversation with me, and it apparently is unchanged over the course of time, despite treatment with five bottles of cough syrup and three bottles of antibiotics.

She is currently producing yellow-tinged sputum approximately 2 to 3 tbsp per day. The patient has also noted chest pain off and on over the last 3 to 4 months in the left parasternal region. It is intermittently worse with motion. She attributes the pain to arthritis. She is also bothered with arthritis in the shoulder on the right as well as on her fingers.

PHYSICAL EXAMINATION: Alert, cooperative, white woman in no acute stress. B/P 152/94. Wt 146. R 18. P 74. Skin warm and dry. Head: no depressions or scalp lesions. Eyes: PERRLA. Fundoscopic exam unremarkable. ENT: clear. Neck: supple, no adenopathy. Carotids equal bilaterally without bruits. Chest: symmetrical. Lungs clear to auscultation and percussion. Heart: no murmur or gallop. Abdomen: no hepato or splenomegaly. Pulses intact. Extremities: no clubbing, cyanosis, or edema. Neurological exam within normal limits.

In view of this lady's chronic cough and right lower lobe collapse, I concur with your suggestion that she may have an endobronchial lesion requiring investigation.

She is scheduled for a fiberoptic bronchoscopy as an outpatient at Methodist Hospital on Tuesday of next week.

Evaluation of Medical Report 6–4: Pleural Atelectasis

1. Was her headache on one side only?

2. Where was the headache localized?

3. Where was her chest pain?

4. Was her liver smaller than normal?

Unit 7 Endocrine and Nervous System

The following medical reports are related to the medical specialties called endocrinology and neurology.

Medical Report 7–1: Microfollicular Adenoma, Hypothyroidism

Dictionary Exercise

Underline the following terms in this report. Use a medical dictionary and Appendix E, "Abbreviations," to write a definition of each word and abbreviation. This exercise helps you to master the terminology in this report.

adenoma_____
auscultation_____
carcinoma_____
cervical_____
clubbing_____
cm_____
edema_____
exophthalmia_____
gravid_____
hepato_____
hirsutism_____
hypothyroidism_____
lymphadenopathy_____
microfollicular_____
percussion_____
pretibial_____
splenomegaly_____
thyroiditis_____
thyroxine_____
tracheal_____

Medical Report 7–1: Microfollicular Adenoma, Hypothyroidism

Read the medical report out loud.

This 31-year-old married mexican woman apparently had developed thyroid disease in 1986. At that time she visited her Mexican physician for evaluation of some changes in hair distribution, including hirsutism of the chin and nipples and decreasing scalp hair.

On physical examination she is a neatly groomed, healthy-appearing woman. The pupils are equal and reactive to light and accommodation. There is mild exophthalmia of the left eye. The thyroid presents as a tiny ½-cm nodule along the lateral aspect of the left lower lobe. Otherwise, the thyroid is small and unremarkable feeling. There is no tracheal deviation or cervical lymphadenopathy. The lungs are clear to percussion and auscultation. The abdomen is gravid. No hepato or splenomegaly. Extremities are free of clubbing or edema. There is no pretibial myxedema.

The recent lab panel shows that she is not getting quite enough thyroxine. It would be nice to get records from her previous physician to see how severe her hypothyroidism was. I answered her many questions about maternal fetal thyroid relationships. She was concerned about cretinism and the baby's health in general.

IMPRESSIONS: Microfollicular adenoma of the left lobe of the thyroid gland in a setting of hypothyroidism, possible chronic thyroiditis; rule out malignant follicular carcinoma.

Evaluation of Medical Report 7–1: Microfollicular Adenoma, Hypothyroidism

1. Are the pupils the same size?

2. Is there any bulging of the eyes?

3. What is a nodule?

4. Refer to Figure 7–1, Locations of Many Endocrine Glands (textbook), to describe exactly where you would palpate the nodule.

5. What is cretinism?

6. What is an adenoma?

7. Is this patient pregnant?

8. What is a lab panel?

9. Is her thyroid gland overactive?

10. Is her liver enlarged?

11. What kind of tumor was revealed?

Medical Report 7–2: Hyperparathyroidism and Diabetes Mellitus

Dictionary Exercise

Underline the following terms in this report. Use a medical dictionary and Appendix E, "Abbreviations," to write a definition of each word and abbreviation. This exercise helps you to master the terminology in this report.

adenoma_____

claudication_____

diabetes mellitus_____

endocrinologist_____

hypercalciuria_____

hyperparathyroidsm_____

osteoarthritis_____

parathyroid_____

retromanubrial region_____

vascular_____

Medical Report 7–2: Hyperparathyroidism and Diabetes Mellitus

Read the medical report out loud.

The patient is a 66-year-old woman who is under evaluation for hyperparathyroidism. Surgery evidently has been recommended, but there is confusion about its urgency. She also has a 14-year-history of type I diabetes mellitus, shoulder pain, and osteoarthritis of the spine; an abnormal chest x-ray with a nodule in the retromanubrial region (which appears to be a stable process); a 100-pack-year smoking history, which ended 3½ years ago; and peripheral vascular disease with claudication.

This former blackjack dealer states her first knowledge of parathyroid disease was about 1990, when the laboratory findings revealed an elevated calcium level. This subsequently led to the diagnosis of hyperparathyroidism. She was further evaluated by an endocrinologist in the Lake Tahoe area, who determined that she also had hypercalciuria, although there is nothing to suggest a history of kidney stones.

IMPRESSION: Hyperparathyroidism and hypercalciuria, probably a parathyroid adenoma.

Evaluation of Medical Report 7–2: Hyperparathyroidism and Diabetes Mellitus

1. Refer to Figure 7–1, The Glands of the Endocrine System (textbook), to designate the location of the parathyroid glands?

2. How many parathyroid glands are there?

3. What is an adenoma?

4. Review Figure 8–1, Anterior View of the Skeleton (textbook), to locate the sternum. In which part of the sternum did the x-ray reveal a nodule?

5. What caused her claudication?

6. What body systems were involved in her condition?

7. Define endocrinologist.

8. What is hypercalciuria?

Medical Report 7–3: Addison's Disease

Dictionary Exercise

Underline the following terms in this report. Use a medical dictionary and Appendix E, "Abbreviations," to write a definition of each word and abbreviation. This exercise helps you to master the terminology in this report.

adrenocortical_____
androgen_____
anorexia_____
arteriosclerotic_____
bid _____
catabolic_____
chronic_____
endocrinologist_____
hypergonadism_____
hyperpigmentation_____
hypogonadism_____

hypothyroidsim_____

insufficiency_____

libido_____

osteoporosis_____

parentally_____

supraphysiologic_____

testosterone_____

Medical Report 7–3: Addison's Disease

The patient relates that shortly after he was married, he became ill with anorexia, weight loss, weakness, and hyperpigmentation of the skin. He became so ill that at the time of hospitalization he was unable to get out of the car to enter the institution. A diagnosis of Addison's disease was made, and he had a dramatic recovery when treated with cortisone. Within a year he was clinically cushingoid, and the dose was reduced. Within 2 years of the onset of his treatment he had his first hip surgery on the left. It is not clear to me what happened, whether this was a fracture or aseptic necrosis, but he had a left hip replacement. He is in the habit of taking 5 mg of prednisone in the morning and 2.5 mg sometime between dinner and bedtime everyday.

It should be noted that he was started on sodium fluoride treatment, apparently for osteoporosis, at just about the same time (perhaps 1963) by doctors in Cincinnati. He has been taking one capsule bid now for some 29 years. It is of interest that he had to have a revision of his left hip reconstruction in 1970, and later in 1970 he required a reconstruction of the left hip, and that apparently is a total hip replacement. He has now been admitted for a right total hip revision and replacement, and he will need to have the left one done before long as well.

From an endocrine standpoint, his case is further complicated by the fact that he was diagnosed as having hypogonadism and hypothyroidism at the same time back in 1960. He does not give a good presentation of symptoms for hypergonadism, relating that he was not aware of having any problems with sex function. He was a young man at the time and would have noticed. He was treated with methyltestosterone. He does not know the dose, but he took it as a pill and went on to take it until 4 years ago, when it was stopped by an endocrinologist. Since that time he has not taken androgen replacement. Since then he has experienced some loss of libido but has no loss of hair, muscle mass, strength or reduction in his normally high energy, ambitious, almost workaholic attitude, according to his wife's description.

IMPRESSIONS:
1. Chronic adrenocortical insufficiency (Addison's disease)
2. Primary hypothyroidism
3. Supposed diagnosis of primary hypogonadis
4. Supposed osteoporosis
5. Arteriosclerotic heart disease, status post–coronary artery bypass graft

COMMENT: There are many issues in this case. Although the diagnosis of Addison's disease is probably correct, I do not believe that prednisone is the correct agent to use. This man should be on hydrocortisone, because I believe that prednisone has more catabolic qualities and is more likely to cause osteoporosis than physiologic doses of hydrocortisone. For the time being we are going to cover him with hydrocortisone, initially parentally, and then we will follow up with an oral dosage while he is in the hospital in supraphysiologic but declining doses. For now we will continue the Florinef because it seems to be serving him well. I told him to discontinue sodium fluoride. He has been taking 88 mg now for 25 and possibly 30 years; that is way more experience than anything that has ever been published, and it is appropriate to discontinue this drug at the present time. His thyroid will be checked as well as his testosterone. He has not taken any androgen replacement, and we do not even know if he needs it. That will be checked.

Evaluation of Medical Report 7–3: Addison's Disease

1. Addison's disease is due to deficiency of which endocrine organ?

2. Did this patient have the usual clinical manifestations of Addison's disease? What are they?

3. Did the endocrinologist suspect that his prednisone therapy might have something to do with his osteoporosis?

4. Which endocrine glands are being treated in his situation?

5. Did he take prednisone for the usual length of time?

6. How was the hydrocortisone initially administered?

7. Was more than the usual dose given because he was hospitalized and could be observed more carefully?

Medical Report 7–4: Alcoholic Admission

Dictionary Exercise

Underline the following terms in this report. Use a medical dictionary and Appendix E, "Abbreviations," to write a definition of each word and abbreviation. This exercise helps you to master the terminology in this report.

adrenocortical_____

androgen_____

anorexia_____

arteriosclerotic_____

bid_____

catabolic_____

chronic_____

cushingoid_____

endocrinologist_____

hypergonadism_____

hyperpigmentation_____

hypogonadism_____

hypothyroidsim_____

insufficiency_____

libido_____

mg_____

Medical Report 7–4: Alcoholic Admission

<u>PRESENT ILLNESS</u>: This 45-year-old white man was admitted to Betty Ford Clinic on 1-14-91 because of uncontrolled fits. The patient has a long medical history that includes bilateral past surgeries for carcinoma 15 to 20 years ago, with no evidence of recurrence. She has also had several skin cancers that required removal and has a long history of alcoholism.

She has recently begun to drink rather regularly again. She has over the past 8 to 9 days become progressively more difficult to handle and has had several grand mal–type seizures. She was brought in to the emergency department and admitted for therapy and evaluation. The patient was seen in neurology consultation, and it was the neurologist's opinion that the patient showed evidence of early Korsakoff psychosis and that her seizure disorder was secondary to her chronic alcoholism.

She was started on thiamine and began to show progressive improvement mentally, though slow. Her affect was inappropriately pleasant and flat, with very little evidence of emotional reaction or awareness of what was happening. The patient was not well oriented to time but did seem to be reasonably oriented to place and persons.

She was uncharacteristically cooperative. In the latter part of her hospital stay, arrangements were made for her to be seen at the alcohol clinic for counseling, which she had previously refused.

On the 14th of February when she was to have been seen, she suddenly returned to her old self and adamantly refused to undertake any sort of alcohol control program, stating that she could take care of it by herself, a fact which she has spent her entire life disproving. She was at that time ambulatory and able to take care of herself and was therefore discharged home with the instruction to pursue outpatient follow-up. She was informed that unless she had some sort of help and was able to remain free of alcohol, her prognosis was poor.

In the hospital she was shown to have some hepatomegaly and moderate elevation of alkaline phosphatase, SGPT and SGOT.

FINAL DIAGNOSES:
1. Chronic alcoholism with malnutrition
2. Seizure disorder secondary to No. 1
3. Chronic liver disease secondary to No. 1
4. Anemia, normocytic, secondary to No. 1

Evaluation of Medical Report 7–4: Alcoholic Admission

1. Did this patient have a history of cancer?

2. What type of seizure disorder does she suffer from?

3. What caused her hepatomegaly?

4. Why is she diagnosed with malnutrition?

Unit 8 Musculoskeletal System

The following medical reports are from orthopedics and physical medicine and rehabilitation. The physicians specializing in this area are known as orthopedist and physiatrist.

Medical Report 8-1: EMG Report on a Status Post–Carpal Tunnel Release

Dictionary Exercise

Underline the following terms in this report. Use a medical dictionary and Appendix E, "Abbreviations," to write a definition of each word and abbreviation. This exercise helps you to master the terminology in this report.

amplitude_____
brachioradialis_____
brevis_____
C7_____
carpal tunnel_____
denervation_____
digit_____
distal_____
dorsal_____
electrodiagnostic_____
interosseous_____
latency_____
median_____
paraspinal_____
peripheral_____
polyphasia_____
syndrome_____
triceps_____

Medical Report 8-1: EMG Report on a Status Post–Carpal Tunnel Release

Read the medical report out loud.

HISTORY: The patient has a history of having a left ulnar transposition and left median carpal tunnel release approximately 3 years ago. She has had recurrence of symptoms since July of last year: worsening in numbness and pain in the medial aspect of the left hand, also involving the third digit.

<u>PHYSICAL EXAMINATION</u>: She has reduced brachioradialis reflex and triceps reflex on the left when compared to the right. Strength is within normal limits.

<u>NERVE CONDUCTION FINDINGS</u>: The nerve conduction studies are all within normal limits, except that the difference between the median and ulnar F wave is borderline, which may be associated with slightly longer distal latency in the median motor conduction.

<u>EMG FINGINGS</u>: There is a trace of spontaneous activity in the C7, C6, and C8 areas of the cervical paraspinal musculature. No other spontaneous activity is recorded in the left abductor pollicis brevis and the first dorsal interosseous, with slight to 1+ polyphasia brevis. There is also slightly increased amplitude in the abductor pollicis brevis when compared to normal.

<u>IMPRESSION</u>:
1. No evidence of acute carpal tunnel syndrome.
2. No evidence of acute ulnar neuropathy at the elbow.
3. Mild electrodiagnostic evidence of left C6-7 denervation in the neck.
4. The possibility of old carpal tunnel syndrome and old ulnar neuropathy exists with the distal reduced recruitment patterns versus a chronic mild radicular problem.
5. No evidence of peripheral neuropathy on electrodiagnostic studies.

Evaluation of Medical Report 8-1: EMG Report on a Status Post-Carpal Tunnel Release

1. With the patient's hand in the anatomic position, refer to Figure 8-1 (textbook), locate the lower arm bone that involves the medial aspect.

2. Is the ring finger or middle finger involved?

3. Is the patient's current discomfort due to acute carpal tunnel syndrome?

4. Does the patient's ring finger straighten out within the normal time frame?

5. Did the electrodiagnostic studies identify any functional disturbances of the peripheral nervous system?

Medical Report 8–2: Lumbosacral Strain

Dictionary Exercise

Underline the following terms in this report. Use a medical dictionary and Appendix E, "Abbreviations," to write a definition of each word and abbreviation. This exercise helps you to master the terminology in this report.

antalgic_____

bilateral_____

extension_____

facet_____

flexion_____

gait_____

hyperextension_____

L5_____

lateral_____

lordotic_____

lumbosacral_____

lumbosacral_____

paresthesia_____

PT_____

S1_____

spondylitic_____

steroid_____

syndrome_____

Medical Report 8-2: Lumbosacral Strain

Read the medical report out loud.

HISTORY OF PRESENT ILLNESS: The patient is seen today for a second opinion regarding a lower back injury. The patient states he injured himself on November 20, 19XX while leaning over and carrying a pallet of frozen pies. He apparently had to move 35 pallets, requiring bending and lifting of pallets of frozen pies, when he experienced some discomfort in his lower back. He states he had a similar injury a couple of years ago, which responded to conservative therapy. The patient has had some gradual improvement with PT, but because of persistent symptoms, was referred to Dr. Gylys for further treatment. Dr. Gylys continued the patient's light duty status and non-steroidal medication after diagnosing bilateral L5-S1 facet syndrome and recommended facet injections.

The patient is here today requesting a second opinion regarding facet injections. He has lower back pain, primarily on the right, which increases with prolonged sitting or bending and occasionally with sneezing. His pain is not increased by hyperextension of his back. He experiences no pain, numbness, or paresthesia in the lower extremities.

REVIEW OF SYSTEMS: Essentially negative.

PHYSICAL EXAMINATION: Lumbosacral: Inspection of gait is normal and non-antalgic. Inspection of lumbosacral spine reveals no loss of normal lordotic curvature. There are no spondylitic deformities present.

Range of motion: Range of motion of forward flexion is 50% of normal. Extension is 100% of normal. Lateral flexion bilaterally is 100% of normal, with the exception of some limitation to the left.

IMPRESSION: Lumbosacral strain.

Evaluation of Medical Report 8-2: Lumbosacral Strain

1. What is the difference between a strain and a sprain?

2. Refer to Figure 8-6 (textbook) and determine if the strain is at the proximal or distal end of the vertebral column?

3. When the patient walked, did he appear to be in pain?

4. Were the lumbar vertebrae curved anteriorly or posteriorly?

5. Is the patient's range of motion the same laterally?

Unit 9 Cardiovascular and Lymphatic Systems

The following medical reports are related to the medical specialty called cardiology and vascular surgery.

Medical Report 9–1: Congestive Heart Failure (CHF)

Dictionary Exercise

Underline the following terms in this report. Use a medical dictionary and Appendix E, "Abbreviations," to write a definition of each word and abbreviation. This exercise helps you to master the terminology in this report.

anemia_____
aspiration_____
CHF_____
constellation_____
CT scan_____
edema_____
endoscopy_____
erythroid_____
hepatosplenomegaly_____
hgb_____
hypochromic_____
lymphocytosis_____
megakaryocytes_____
microcytic_____
myeloid_____
pitting_____
pleurisy_____

Medical Report 9–1: Congestive Heart Failure (CHF)

Read the medical report out loud.

The patient presents with a 3- to 4-month history of recurrent shortness of breath, as well as recurrent chest pressure. The patient was in her usual state of health when she developed the progressive onset of shortness of breath to the point where she was unable to perform her activities of daily living. The symptoms were described as intermittent shortness of breath, which at first was unrelated to exertion and typically made better by rest. The patient's history of chest discomfort is remarkable for a chest heaviness/pressure, which radiates to her upper chest and neck, lasting 5 to 10 minutes and, again, not necessarily related to exertion. She has not noted any overt pleurisy.

While in the emergency department, she was documented as having an hgb of 6.2, with an hct of 20.1, and also noted to have 3+ pitting edema, as well as overt CHF. She was seen by her family practice physician who felt that the constellation of findings was quite dramatic, and she required inpatient therapy.

As an inpatient she received IV Lasix as well as potassium supplementation, and her smear was reviewed, documentating hypochromic microcytic anemia. She was seen in consultation by a cardiologist, who recommended transfusion, as well as extensive upper endoscopy, which is planned for tomorrow.

OF NOTE: She has had a history of anemia and has been seen in consultation in the past. A bone marrow aspiration revealed adequate cellularity and normal numbers of megakaryocytes. No abnormalities of the erythroid or myeloid series. There was decreased bone marrow iron, and there was lymphocytosis. Interestingly, she was believed to have hepatosplenomegaly by CT scan, but nuclear evaluation failed to reveal this.

ASSESSMENT:
1. Congestive heart failure, most likely on the basis of both severe anemia and probably intrinsic heart disease, exacerbated by the anemia
2. Severe iron deficiency anemia, with etiology unclear at present but currently under evaluation
3. Chronic venous stasis in the lower extremities
4. Evidence of mild peripheral vascular disease by examination.
5. Hypertension, currently in need of control
6. Status post release of Dupuytren's contracture of the right hand several months ago
7. History of splenomegaly and anemia, without etiologic diagnosis in 1986

Evaluation of Medical Report 9–1: Congestive Heart Failure (CHF)

1. Was the patient constantly short of breath?

2. Was her hemoglobin within the normal range when checked in the ED?

3. What is the normal range for hemoglobin and hematocrit values?

4. What type of anemia did the patient have?

5. What is pitting edema?

6. What type of examination did the cardiologist recommend?

7. What organs appeared enlarged by CT scan?

Medical Report 9–2: Acute Inferolateral Myocardial Infarction

Dictionary Exercise

Underline the following terms in this report. Use a medical dictionary and Appendix E, "Abbreviations," to write a definition of each word and abbreviation. This exercise helps you to master the terminology in this report.

acute_____

bradycardia_____

coronary_____

diaphoresis_____

EKG_____

infarction_____

inferolateral_____

ischemia_____

MI_____

myocardial_____

sublingual_____

substernal_____

tachycardia_____

Medical Report 9–2: Acute Inferolateral Myocardial Infarction

Read the medical report out loud.

The patient is an 84-year-old hispanic woman with coronary artery disease, status post–inferior wall MI in 1991, status post Code Blue for ventricular tachycardia associated with the inferior wall MI, who now presents with chest pain X 3 hours.

This morning she developed a sharp substernal heaviness that was 10/10 with no associated nausea, vomiting, shortness of breath, or diaphoresis. The patient received two sublingual nitroglycerins in the ambulance and had some improvement of her chest pain.

The first EKG on arrival to the emergency room showed an old inferior wall myocardial infarction that was similar to her previous EKG. The EKG in the ED showed changes consistent with inferolateral ischemia versus MI. She had one episode of junctional bradycardia with a new left bundle branch block that resolved after one dose of atropine.

Initial EKG showed a normal sinus rhythm at a rate of 75, left axis deviation at –30 degrees; intervals are normal. There were large Q's in leads III and aVF. Poor R-wave progression, flattened T's, unchanged from 09/92. The second EKG showed sinus bradycardia at a rate of 55, left axis deviation of –1 degree, QRS widened to 0.12, and there were less than 1-mm ST elevations in leads I, aVL, V4-V6, as well as II and III. The T waves were up laterally.

Evaluation of Medical Report 9–2: Acute Inferolateral Myocardial Infarction

1. Was the heaviness above or below the breastbone?

2. Did she break out in "cold sweat"?

3. How was the nitroglycerin administered in the ambulance?

4. While in the ED, an EKG showed a decrease in blood supply to which coronary arteries?

5. Refer to Fgure 9–5 and notice the normal EKG pattern described by the physician for the patient..

Medical Report 9–3: Left Foot Ischemic Lesions

Dictionary Exercise

Underline the following terms in this report. Use a medical dictionary and Appendix E, "Abbreviations," to write a definition of each word and abbreviation. This exercise helps you to master the terminology in this report.

angioplasty_____
bilaterally_____
brachials_____
carotids_____
digits_____
dorsalis_____
dorsum_____
femorals bruits_____
ischemic_____
lesions_____

occlusive_____

pedis_____

popliteal_____

radials_____

ruborous_____

superficial_____

tibials_____

trifurcation_____

ulceration_____

Medical Report 9–3: Left Foot Ischemic Lesions

HISTORY: The patient was admitted for pancreatic symptoms; however, it was noted that her right foot had ischemic-appearing lesions. The patient said her foot was very painful a number of days ago, but the pain has resolved since taking Coumadin. She denied any previous surgeries to her arteries and/or veins, and she denied any previous episodes of similar phenomenon.

EXTREMITIES: Her upper extremities appeared normal to gross evaluation. Her lower extremities: The left leg was cooler than the right, and there was ruborous discoloration to the dorsum of the foot and the second and third toes, with no frank ulceration at the digits; however, on the dorsum of the foot there was a small healing scab without any signs of infection. The patient's superficial venous system appeared adequate.

PULSES: Radials: 3+ and 3+. Brachials: 3+ and 3+. There was a loop forearm graft in the left forearm with a good thrill. Carotids: 3+ and 3+ without bruits. Her femorals were 3+ and 3+, and bruits were noted bilaterally. The right popliteal was trace, left was absent. The right dorsalis pedis was trace, the left was absent. Posterior tibials were absent bilaterally.

IMPRESSION: She has near-ischemic ulceration or severe ischemia at present to her right foot with suspected superficial femoral artery, as well as trifurcation occlusive disease.

RECOMMENDATIONS: Baseline noninvasive studies and angiography. It is hoped that an angioplasty will resolve her ischemic lesions; if not, bypass surgery should be considered.

Evaluation of Medical Report 9–3: Left Foot Ischemic Lesions

1. What was this patient's circulatory status?

2. Does Coumadin thin or thicken the blood?

3. Was the circulation the same in both legs?

4. Is the dorsum the same as the top side of the foot?

5. What color was her foot and toes?

6. What were the values of the pulses in the lower arm?

7. What was the pulse value behind the left knee?

8. Which foot has the problem?

9. Is the doctor hopeful that surgical repair of the vessel will improve her ischemia?

Medical Report 9–4: Pulmonary Embolus

Dictionary Exercise

Underline the following terms in this report. Use a medical dictionary and Appendix E, "Abbreviations," to write a definition of each word and abbreviation. This exercise helps you to master the terminology in this report.

phlebitis_____
DVT_____
pulmonary embolus_____
GI_____
IV_____
heparin_____
Greenfield filter_____
inferior vena cava_____
cellulitis_____
Ancef_____
pulmonary lung scan_____
anticoagulation_____
Asacol_____
Coumadin_____

pro-time_____

dx_____

colitis_____

Medical Report 9–4: Pulmonary Embolus

Read the medical report out loud.

A 70-year-old-man was admitted to the hospital with phlebitis to the right upper extremity, DVT to the left lower extermity, and pulmonary embolus in the left lung field. This gentlemen had been seeing Dr. Lemp for a GI bleed and was placed on medications. He suddenly developed the DVT in the left lower extremity. He has never had this problem before. On hospital admission he was placed on IV heparin. In consultation with Dr. Yovon, we determined it appropriate to place a Greenfield filter in his inferior vena cava, which was done without complications. While in the hospital the patient had been placed on IV Ancef for his phlebitis and cellulitis to the right upper extremity. These have cleared, as has the pain and discomfort to his left lower leg. A pulmonary lung scan repeated yesterday shows no change, but considering his age, it's felt that it may take months for there to be good resolution. The patient's pro-time on discharge is 15, which is where it should be. Some low-dose anticoagulation should work well with his Greenfield filter.

The patient is discharged today and is instructed to continue his Ascol 800 mg. daily, which was given to him for his bowels. He's placed on Coumadin 2 mg daily. He will have his pro-times checked twice a week.

He will see me in about 10 days. Dr. Yovon will see him in 1 month. He's advised to call sooner if there are any problems.

Final discharge dx: phlebitis to right upper extremity resolved; DVT to left lower extremity resolved; pulmonary embolism left lung field; colitis.

Evaluation of Medical Report 9–4: Pulmonary Embolus

1. What is the dangerous complication of a DVT that happened to this patient?

2. What is the purpose of a Greenfield filter?

3. What are the anticoagulant medications prescribed to this patient?

4. Why is it important for the patient to have his pro-times checked twice a week after discharge?

Unit 10 Special Senses: The Eyes and Ears

The following medical reports are related to the medical specialty called otolaryngology (ENT), plastic surgery, and ophthalmology. The physicians are called otolaryngolists, plastic surgeons, and ophthalmologists.

Medical Report 10-1: Nasal Deformity

Dictionary Exercise

Underline the following terms in this report. Use a medical dictionary and Appendix E, "Abbreviations," to write a definition of each word and abbreviation. This exercise helps you master the terminology in this report.

adherent_____
cartilage_____
columella_____
concha_____
dissection_____
dorsum_____
graft_____
hemostasis_____
impregnated_____
infiltration_____
intracartilaginous_____
intransal_____
intravenous_____
lateral_____
longitudinal_____
nasal_____
postauricular_____
subperichondrial_____
sutures_____

Medical Report 10-1: Nasal Deformity

OPERATION: Removal of old cartilage graft and replacement with new cartilage graft, dorsum of nose.

<u>FINDINGS</u>: The patient is a white male who has a cartilage graft that seems to be absorbing in an irregular manner and thus producing external appearance deformities. He is now admitted for removal of as much of the old cartilage graft as possible and insertion of new cartilage graft.

<u>PROCEDURE</u>: The patient received intravenous droperidol, Ativan, morphine, and Versed. Xylocaine 1% with epinephrine and Neutracaine was used for local infiltration around the perimeter of the nose. Normal saline was injected across the dorsum and under the very thin skin around the cartilage graft. Soft cotton impregnated with 10% cocaine and Adrenalin was inserted in both nostrils and left in place for 10 minutes. On the right side, an intracartilaginous incision was made and extended down the columella and, careful and sharp dissection was used to open up the pocket across the dorsum of the nose and around the cartilage graft. The graft was densely adherent to the dorsum of extremely thin skin, so it was impractical to remove it as a unit. It was divided into multiple pieces and either repositioned or removed in this manner leaving the attached portion to the skin in its position. The pocket was adequate and hemostasis was well controlled. On the left ear, a postauricular incision was made and the concha exposed. An incision was made in the concha and a subperichondrial excision carried out. Hemostasis was meticulously controlled. The graft was taken in longitudinal pieces and layering carried out in order to extend the length and thickness in the appropriate areas. This was all done with interrupted 5-0 Vicryl sutures. Once the graft had been measured, it was inserted without any trauma. The portion of the graft extending across the nasal bones was purposely left wide, and a longitudinal incision made on the dorsal aspect on both sides so that the lateral portions of the graft would fold down. This fit in and gave a smooth contour to the dorsum. The intranasal wounds were closed with interrupted chromic catgut. Loose taping across the dorsum was carried out, and no other pressure placed on the skin. The patient tolerated the procedure well.

Evaluation of Medical Report 10-1: Nasal Deformity

1. Why is the patient having the graft replaced?

2. How was the patient's operative medication administered?

3. In which nostril did the doctor create the first incision?

4. Where did the doctor take the graft from to replace the defective nasal graft?

Medical Report 10–2: Relative Microgenia

Dictionary Exercise

Underline the following terms in this report. Use a medical dictionary and Appendix E, "Abbreviations," to write a definition of each word and abbreviation. This exercise helps you to master the terminology in this report.

augmentation_____
bilateral_____
frenulum_____
intraoral_____
mentoplasty_____
microgenia_____
mm_____
mucosa_____
osseous_____
subperiosteal_____
supine_____

Medical Report 10–2: Relative Microgenia

OPERATION: Augmentation mentoplasty, intraoral approach.

SUMMARY: The patient was taken to the operating room where she was placed on the table in the supine position. She was prepped and draped in the customary sterile fashion. The chin was anesthetized by bilateral mental nerve blocks with ¼ % Marcaine with epinephrine, 1:200,000, followed by local infiltration in the area of implantation. After a suitable time the frenulum was tattooed with gential violet, and an 18-mm intraoral incision was made. An adequate cuff of mucosa and muscle was left for layered closure subsequent to implant placement. Approximately 1 cm below the mucosal incision, the dissection was diverted to the osseous level, where subperiosteal dissection was carried out with a Joseph elevator along the inferior margin of the mandible, creating a pock corresponding to that marked on the skin using the implant as a template. The implant was inserted easily and found to lie naturally in a symmetricalal fashion. Closure was then obtained with one 4-0 Vicryl placed through the central portion of the implant and then to midline muscle along the superior process. Additional closure was carried out in muscle with a 4-0 Dexon in two layers, followed by interrupted 5-0 Vicryl careful closure of the mucosa, producing an essentially watertight seal. The chin was then dressed with elastic ½-inch Steri-strips.

Evaluation of Medical Report 10–2: Relative Microgenia

1. Was the patient lying on her side?

2. What was wrong with the patient's chin?

3. What was done to correct the problem?

4. Was the incision made inside the mouth or between the structure connecting the lip and the gums?

5. What type of instrument was used to dissect the periosteum from the mandible?

6. Were individual stitches taken to close the mucosa?

Medical Report 10–3: Cataract, Left Eye

Dictionary Exercise

Underline the following terms in this report. Use a medical dictionary and Appendix E, "Abbreviations," to write a definition of each word and abbreviation. This exercise helps you to master the terminology in this report.

anterior_____

aphakic_____

cataract_____

corneal_____

cryoextraction_____

extraction_____

intracapsular_____

iridotomy_____

iris_____

lumbus_____

peripheral_____

peritomy_____

pupil_____

speculum_____

vitreous_____

Medical Report 10-3: Cataract, Left Eye

OPERATION: Intracapsular cataract extraction and peripheral iridotomy times ii, left eye.

PROCEDURE: After routine sterile preparation and draping under local anesthesia, a lid speculum was placed between the lids of the left eye, which was then turned downward with a blue superior rectus stay suture of 6-0 black silk. Peritomy was made from 8:45 to 3:15 o'clock, and a groove was made in the surgical lumbus from 2:45 counterclockwise to 9:15 o'clock. A 6-0 black silk mattress suture was placed across the wound at 12 o'clock and pulled aside. The anterior chamber was entered at 10:30 o'clock with a microsharp blade, and then an incision was made from 10:30 to 1:15 o'clock.

The incision was then extended through the groove from 9:15 to 2:45 o'clock, using right and left hand corneal scissors. Peripheral iridotomies were performed at 11 and 1 o'clock positions. Iris was pulled aside and anterior surface of lens dried with Weck sponge. The posterior chamber was irrigated with 1:7000 solution of alpha-chymotrypsin through iridotomies and posterior iris below.

Cryoextraction was placed on the lens at 12 o'clock, just anterior to the equator, and the lens forwarded and intact and entered without loss of vitreous. The preplaced mattress suture was pulled up, tightened as a mattress suture. The anterior chamber was irrigated with Miochol in order to bring the pupil down and the iris out of the wound.

The wound was further completely closed with interrupted sutures of 8-0 black silk. The anterior chamber was fully reformed to aphakic depth by using interrupted 6-0 plain gut sutures. The eye was dressed with multiple 1% atropine ointment, eye pad, shield, and tape.

Evaluation of Medical Report 10–3: Cataract, Left Eye

1. What is a cataract?

2. What type of instrument did they use to remove the lens?

3. What temperature was it?

4. What does the iris look like?

5. Was the remove the iris?

Answer Key for Evaluation of Medical Reports

Medical Report 2–1: GI Evaluation
1. Refer to Figure 2–1, Digestive System (textbook), to determine where the gallbladder is located in relation to the liver? **Posteriorly and inferiorly**
2. Examine Figure 2–2, Accessory Organs of Digestion (textbook). What duct does the doctor suspect might have retained stones? **Common bile duct**
3. Was her preoperative pain constant? **No, intermittent pain lasting 2 to 4 hours**
4. How does her most recent postoperative episode of discomfort (pain) differ from the initial pain she described? **Continuous deep right-sided pain, which took a cresdcendo pattern**
5. Has she had any other surgeries of the GI system? **Yes**
6. If so, what were they? If not, which systems were involved? **Tonsillectomy, appendectomy, and cholecystectomy**
7. Were the laboratory findings within normal limits? **Yes**
8. There is the possibility of an ulcer. Refer to Figure 2–1, Digestive System (textbook), to determine which part of the bowel is involved? Is this the most common site?
Duodenum, yes
9. What x-ray showed no abnormalities? **Upper GI**
10. What structures are examined in an upper GI? Refer to Appendix C, "Radiographic Procedures," barium swallow. **Esophagus, stomach, and duodenum**

Medical Report 2–2: Operative Report—Left Colon Resection
1. Refer to Figure 2–1, Digestive System (textbook), to identify the location of the lesion. **Located in the patient's upper left quadrant at the splenic flexure.**
2. Describe the shape of the lesion. **Round (ring shaped).**
3. Was the lesion benign or malignant? **Malignant.**
4. Did the lesion spread to the liver? **No (without hepatic metastasis).**
5. The doctor did a colocolostomy. What is the difference between that and a colostomy?
A new opening was created between the segments of the large bowel that were removed, rather than to the outside surface.
6. Is the greater curvature on the lateral or the medial side of the stomach? **Lateral.**
7. What is an anastomosis? **A communication between two structures.**
8. What are vital signs? **Blood pressure, temperature, pulse, and respirations.**

Medical Report 2–3: Colonoscopy and Polypectomy
1. What is the difference between a sessile polyp and a pedunculated polyp?
2. **A sessile polyp is attached at a base; a pedunculated polyp has a stemlike stalk.**
3. How many sessile polyps did the patient have? **Four.**
4. Was the endoscope advanced into the small bowel? **Yes** If so, into which part of the small bowel? **Terminal ileum.**
5. As the endoscope was being removed, a well-defined semipedunculated polyp was identified. How far into the bowel was it located? **16 cm.**
6. What is a diverticulum? **Outpouching of the structure.**

7. This patient had one or two diverticular openings. In which part of the large bowel were they identified? **Transverse colon.**
8. Why did the doctor recommend annual colonoscopy? **Family history and multiplicity of polyps.**

Medical Report 3–1: Nephrology Consultation

1. Were the results of the preoperative BUN and creatinine studies abnormal? **Yes**
2. What organ function is evaluated with those laboratory tests? **Kidney**
3. What is an IVP? **X-ray demonstrating kidney (execretory) function**
4. Why has his skin turgor decreased? **Dehydration and age**
5. Has the patient experienced any decrease in urinary output?
Slight decrease in urinary output
6. Where is the right hypochondriac region? **Below the right rib cage**
7. What is ascites? **Accumulation of fluid in the peritoneal cavity**
8. Did the patient have any swelling of the extremities? **No**
9. Which part of the kidney has inflammation? **Renal pelvis**

Medical Report 3–2 Probable Urosepsis

Do you suppose the vaginitis is a complication from taking ampicillin? Check with a *Physician's Desk Reference* for side effects of this drug. **Yes, monialial infections**
Did the vaginal discharge consist of pus? **Yes, purulent vaginal drainage**
What caused her pulmonary embolism? **Clots in the leg**
Did she have any enlargements of the abdominal organs? **No**
How did they hydrate her? **Intravenous fluids with antibiotics**
Was her white count significant? **Yes, 12.1**
Was the specific gravity within normal limits? **Yes, 1.025**

Medical Report 3–3: Ureteral Calculus

1. What caused the ureteral obstruction? **Calculus (stones).**
2. What is a cystoscope? **Instrument used for examining the bladder.**
3. What is the difference between a retrograde pyelogram and an IVP?
In a retrograde pyelogram, dye is instilled through the ureteral catheters to visualize the kidneys; in an IVP, the dye is injected intravenously.
4. Why was the urologist unable to remove the ureteral calculus?
The middle portion of the ureter has numerous strictures and narrow areas, and it is impossible to pass the rigid scope beyond this point.
5. Which part of the ureter was obstructed? **Mid ureter.**
6. What is a stent? **A mold to provide support for the tubular structure.**
7. How many scopes did the doctor use? **Four.** Name them? **Cystoscope, ureteroscope, flexible French scope, and rigid uteroscope.**
8. Did the radiolucent object appear white or dark on the x-ray? **White.**

Medical Report 4–1: Redundant Facial and Neck Skin with Submental Adipose Tissue
1. Did they make an incision under the chin?
Yes, a 0.5-cm incision was made in the submental crease.
2. What method did they use to control bleeding? **electrocautery**
3. Where is the tragus located? **In front of the ear.**
4. What suture did they use to close behind the ear? **5-0 Vicryl**

Medical Report 4–2: Burn, Right Hand
1. Does the patient have feeling in her hand with the burn?
No, there is anesthesia over the eschar.
2. Is it the back or the palm of the hand that received the burn? **Palm.**
3. Was it her thumb side that was burned? **No, it was the ulnar (little finger) side.**
4. Did the doctor prescribe oral antibiotics? **No, systemic antibiotics were not required.**
5. Did she lose any muscle function? **Not at the time of last visit.**

Medical Report 4–3: Lesion of Left Ring Finger
1. What did the doctor do to the lesion? **Initially, cryotherapy and antibiotics were used, followed by shave biopsy and finally by excisional biopsy.**
2. How long had the patient had the lesion? **Approximately 6 months.**
3. How did the dermatologist treat the lesion initially? **With cryotherapy and antibiotics.**
4. Where did the doctor administer the anesthetic block? **Digital block (with a 2-cc injection of 2% Lodicaine near the neurovascular bundles of the fingers).**
5. How deep did the surgeon cut to remove the lesion? **Below the dermis.**

Medical Report 5-1: Carcinoma, Lower Inner Breast, Clinical Stage 1, Discovered by Mammography
1. Did this patient have symptoms that caused her to seek medical attention? **No.**
2. Was the nodule located above or below the breast? **Below, at the inframammary line.**
3. Could the doctors feel the nodule? **No, it was non-palpable.**
4. Did they treat the nodule with x-ray therapy? **No.**
5. At what age did she start her menses? **11.**
6. At what age did her breast develop? **12.**
7. What is wrong with her eyes? **She has arcus senilus, which is a grey opaque ring surrounding the margin of the cornea.**
8. Are her nipples of normal contour? **Yes, they are everted.**
9. Why did they have her donate a unit of her own blood prior to surgery?
To prevent postoperative residual axillary and subcutaneous flap fluid collection.
10. In which direction is her uterus flexed? **Backward (retroverted).**
11. What is wrong with her feet?
Hallux valgus (angulation of the great toe towards the other toes).

Medical Report 5-2: Bilateral Hypomastia
1. What was wrong with her breasts? **They were small.**
2. What is an augmentation mammoplasty? **Surgical enlargement of the breast.**
3. Where was the incision made? **Around the lower half of the aerola.**
4. Were individual sutures closing the skin used? **Yes, interrupted sutures were made.**

Medical Report 5-3: Breast Reduction
1. How many pregnancies have been successful for this patient? **Two.**
2. What makes this person a good candidate for a reduction mammoplasty?
Pendulous breasts, stable weight after significant loss.
3. Is mammary hypertrophy a familial trait? **Yes.**
4. What symptoms does this patient have involving her fingers due to mammary hypertrophy? **Paraesthesias.**
5. Where is her rash? **In the intertriginous regions. (Where skin surfaces touch other skin surfaces, such as folds of the breasts.)**
6. What is this client's abdominal problem? **She has a large apron of skin as a result of the weight loss.**
7. Does her skin have good turgor? **No, it is severely ptotic (sagging) and lacking in elasticity.**

Medical Report 5-4: Impotence and Penile Prosthesis
1. What was the main reason the patient sought medical help? **Impotence and penile implant.**
2. What medical treatment was given prior to surgery? **Medications for hypertension.**
3. What type of prosthesis did the urologist use? **Flexirod penile prosthesis.**
4. Did the patient have postoperative problems? **No, the procedure was benign.**
5. Did the patient have difficulty walking postoperatively?
No, he was ambulating with no pain.
6. How many times a day did the patient take the antibiotic? **qid, four times a day.**

Medical Report 5-5: Arterial and Venous Leak Impotence
1. What does this gentleman's doctor feel is the source of his problem?
A combination of arterial and venous leak impotence
2. Which part of the extremities demonstrates varicose veins? **Lower legs**
3. Does this patient have a decrease in penile sensation and reflexes? **No**
4. How often does the client have to take Yokon? **Two tablets three times a day**
5. What will the angiodynography prove? **The quality of his vascular status**

Medical Report 6–1: Pulmonary Function Report (Pre- vs Post-comparison)
1. Did this patient have any difficulty in breathing? **Yes**
2. What was the presenting diagnosis? **Shortness of breath**
3. What was the hydrogen ion concentration? **7.38**
4. What was the level of bicarbonate radical? **22**
5. What was the partial pressure of carbon dioxide? (Clue: This patient is retaining carbon dioxide.) **78**

Medical Report 6–2: Left Empyema
1. How was this patient's tuberculosis treated?
Wedge resection in the left upper and lower lobes.
2. What type of cancer did the patient have? **Squamous cell.**
3. Did the patient have any postoperative complications? **No.**
4. What is the difference between sputum and saliva? **Sputum is the abnormal excretion from the lungs and bronchi that usually contains blood, pus, and bacteria, whereas saliva is the clear secretion from salivary glands that moistens the mouth.**
5. Why did the doctor do a needle aspiration?
Patient became feverish and x-rays revealed a new air-filled level in the left thorax.
6. What did the exudate look like? **It was purulent (contained pus, staphyloccal bacteria.)**
7. Did the patient have any sudden shortness of breath at night? **No.**
8. Did the patient have to sleep in a "propped up" position? **No.**
9. When the doctor checked the neurological reflexes of his toes, did they point upward or downward? **Downward (plantar).**
10. If a tube cannot be inserted in the left chest, what will be done to remove the fluid? **Thoractomy.**

Medical Report 6–3: Bronchogenic Carcinoma
1. What two diagnostic procedures were done at the county hospital?
Bronchoscopy and needle biopsy.
2. What complication followed the needle biopsy? **Pneumothorax.**
3. What did they do correct the pneumothorax? **Closed drainage for about 10 days.**
4. Why did they remove the visceral pleura from the right lung?
They did the decortication because she had a spontaneous hemopneumothorax that bled out into the right chest cavity.

Medical Report 6–4: Pleural Atelectasis
1. Was her headache on one side only? **No, it was bitemporal.**
2. Where was the headache localized? **In the temporal area.**
3. Where was her chest pain? **On the left side of the sternum.**
4. Was her liver smaller than normal?
No mention, other than she did not have an enlarged liver.

Medical Report 7–1: Microfollicular Adenoma, Hypothyroidism
1. Are the pupils the same size? **Yes.**
2. Is there any bulging of the eyes? Yes, **mild exophthalmia, left eye.**
3. What is a nodule? **Lump, raised, solid lesion more than 5 mm.**
4. Refer to Figure 7–1, Locations of Many Endocrine Glands (textbook), to describe exactly where you would palpate the nodule. **Outside edge on the left lower part of the thyroid.**
5. What is cretinism? **Result of hypothyroidism in infants, which leads to mental, retardation, impaired growth, low body temperature, and abnormal bone formation.**
6. What is an adenoma? **A benign tumor of a gland.**
7. Is this patient pregnant? **Yes**
8. What is a lab panel? **A series of test performed on a blood sample.**
9. Is her thyroid gland overactive? **No, she has hypothyroidism.**
10. Is her liver enlarged? **No.**
11. What kind of tumor was revealed? **Microfillicular adenoma.**

Medical Report 7–2: Hyperparathyroidism and Diabetes Mellitus
1. Refer to Figure 7–1, The Glands of the Endocrine System (textbook), to designate the location of the parathyroid glands? **The four parathyroid glands are located bilaterally on the thyroid gland.**
2. How many parathyroid glands are there? **Four.**
3. What is an adenoma? **A benign tumor of a gland.**
4. Review to Figure 8–1, Anterior View of the Skeleton (textbook), to locate the sternum. In which part of the sternum did the x-ray reveal a nodule? **Behind the manubrium.**
5. What caused her claudication?
6. **Peripheral vascular disease, probably due to her smoking history.**
7. Which body systems were involved in her condition? **Endocrine, circulatory.**
8. Define endocrinologist.
M.D. who specializes in treating diseases of the endocrine system.
9. What is hypercalciuria? **Excessive amount of calcium in the urine.**

Medical Report 7–3: Addison's Disease
1. Addison's disease is due to deficiency of which endocrine organ? **Adrenal glands**
2. Did this patient have the usual clinical manifestations of Addison's disease? **Yes.** What were they? **Anorexia, weight loss, fatigue (weakness), GI symptoms, hypoglycemia, hypotension, decrease in blood sodium, high serum potassium level**
3. Did the endocrinologist suspect that his prednisone therapy might have something to do with his osteoporosis? **Yes (see comment)**
4. What endocrine glands are being treated in his situation? **Thyroid and adrenal glands**
5. Did he take Prednisone for the usual length of time? **No, much longer**
6. How did they administer the hydrocortisone initially? **Parenterally, by injection**
7. Was more than the usual dose given since he was hospitalized and could be observed more carefully? **Yes, supraphysiological doses**

Medical Report No. 7–4: Alcoholic Admission
1. Did this patient have a history of cancer? **Yes.**
2. What type of seizure did she suffer from? **Grand mal.**
3. What caused her hepatomegaly? **Alcohol.**
4. Why is she diagnosed with malnutrition? **Chronic alcoholism was a contributing factor.**

Medical Report 8–1: EMG Report on a Status Post–Carpal Tunnel Release
1. With the patient's hand in the anatomic position, refer to Figure 8–1 (textbook), locate the lower arm bone that involves the medial aspect? **Ulna**
2. Is the ring finger or middle finger involved? **Middle finger**
3. Is the patient's current discomfort due to acute carpal tunnel syndrome? **Yes**
4. Does the patient's ring finger straighten out within the normal time frame? **No**
5. Did the electrodiagnostic studies identify any functional disturbances of the peripheral nervous system? **A slight increase in amplitude of the abductor pollicis brevis**

Medical Report 8–2: Lumbosacral Strain
1. What is the difference between a strain and a sprain? **A sprain is a wrenching or twisting of a joint with partial rupture of its ligaments. A strain is the overstretching of a muscle.**
2. Looking at Figure 8–6 (textbook), determine whether the strain is at the proximal or distal end of the vertebral column? **Distal (L5-S1).**
3. When the patient walked, did he appear to be in pain? **No.**
4. Were the lumbar vertebrae curved anteriorly or posteriorly? **Anteriorly.**
5. Is the patient's range of motion the same laterally? **Yes.**

Medical Report 9–1: Congestive Heart Failure (CHF)
1. Was the patient constantly short of breath? **No, intermittently.**
2. Was her hemoglobin within the normal range when checked in the ED? **No, it was very low.**
3. What is the normal range for hemoglobin and hematocrit values? **Hemoglobin values vary from 12 to 18 g. Hematocrit values are 42±5, and even lower for females. (Answers will vary depending upon the resource used.)**
4. What type of anemia did the patient have? **Severe iron deficiency anemia**
5. What is pitting edema? **Where the tissues show prolonged indentation when pressure has been applied.**
6. What type of examination did the cardiologist recommend? **Upper endoscopy.**
7. Which organs appeared enlarged on CT scan? **The liver and spleen.**

Medical Report 9–2: Acute Inferolateral Myocardial Infarction
1. Was the heaviness above or below the breastbone? **Below**
2. Did she break out in "cold sweat"? **No diaphoresis**
3. How was nitroglycerin administered in the ambulance? **Sublingually**
4. While in the ED, an EKG showed a decrease in blood supply to which coronary arteries?
   Inferolaterals
5. Refer to Fgure 9–5 and notice the normal EKG pattern desribed by the physician for this patient.

Medical Report 9–3: Left Foot Ischemic Lesions
1. What was this patient's circulatory status? **Poor, she has ischemia.**
2. Does Coumadin thin or thicken the blood? **Thins the blood.**
3. Was the circulation the same in both legs? **No, the left leg is worse than the right.**
4. Is the dorsum the same as the top side of the foot? **Yes.**
5. What color was her foot and toes? **Dark ruby red.**
6. What were the values of the pulses in the lower arm?
7. **Radial and brachial pulses were both assessed at 3+.**
8. What was the pulse value behind the left knee? **The popliteal pulse was absent.**
9. What foot has the problem? **Right**
10. Is the doctor hopeful that surgical repair of the vessel will improve her ischemia?
    Yes, if angioplasty is not successful, then bypass surgery should be considered.

Medical Report 9–4: Pulmonary Embolus
1. What is the dangerous complication of a DVT that happened to this patient?
2. **The DVT may break away and form a pulmonary embolism.**
3. What is the purpose of a Greenfield filter? **It traps large emboli.**
4. What are the anticoagulant medications prescribed to this patient?
   Heparin and Coumadin.
5. Why is it important for the patient to have pro-times checked twice a week after discharge?
   To monitor the side affect of hemorrhage from the anticoagulant medication.

Medical Report 10–1: Nasal Deformity
1. Why is the patient having the graft replaced?
Because it is being absorbed in an irregular manner
2. How was the patient's operative medication administered?
Intravenously and by local infiltration
3. In which nostril did the doctor create the first incision? **Right nostril**
4. Where did the doctor take the graft from to replace the defective nasal graft? **From the left ear**

Medical Report 10–2: Relative Microgenia.
1. Was the patient lying on her side? **No, she was placed on her back.**
2. What was wrong with the patient's chin? **It was small; she had microgenia.**
3. What did they do to correct the problem? **They inserted a prosthesis (implant) below the subperiosteum along the inferior margin of the mandible.**
4. Was the incision made inside the mouth or between the structure connecting the lip and the gums? **Between the lip and the gums.**
5. What type of instrument was used to dissect the periosteum from the mandible?
Joseph periosteal elevator
6. Were individual stitches taken to close the mucosa? **Yes, with interrupted 5-0 Vicryl**

Medical Report 10–3: Cataract, Left Eye
1. What is a cataract? **Opacities that form on the lens or capsule that encloses the lens.**
2. What type of instrument did they use to remove the lens? **A cryoprobe.**
3. What temperature was it? **Cold.**
4. What does the iris look like? **It is the colored portion of the eye.**
5. Did they remove the iris? **No, they did an iridotomy.**

CROSSWORD PUZZLE UNIT 2: DIGESTIVE SYSTEM

Across

1. Instrument to cut the esophagus
7. Pertaining to the stomach
10. How many halves in a football game?
11. Body waste; stool
13. To be the best
14. Meaning of both **-dynia** and **-algia**
15. Prefix meaning under
17. Word root for bladder
18. Suffix meaning abnormal condition
19. Shakespeare's play: _ *You Like It*
20. Abbreviation for registered nurse
21. Health-care professionals use prefixes, combining forms, and suffixes to ___ medical words.
22. This person can't be a chooser.
25. Suffix meaning surgical removal
26. Surgical procedure to form a new opening in the ilium
29. Chronic inflammation of the ileum is known as ____ disease.
31. Relating to the intestines
33. Gangster's gun
35. Not quiet
36. Combining form for tongue
38. Literally, S-shaped; pertaining to the lower part of the descending colon
39. Surgical procedure to form a new opening in the duodenum

Down

1. Combining form for intestines
2. Combining form for the mouth
3. Word root for the liver
4. The three salivary ____ are the submaxillary, sublingual, and parotid.
5. The suffix **-stomy** means forming a new mouth or ____.
6. Ophthalm/o refers to the _____.
7. Abbreviation for gastrointestinal
8. Word root for poison
9. Inflammation of the colon
12. The suffix **-rrhaphy** means to ____.
16. Some physicians record their notes by _____ them into a tape recorder.
19. Suffix meaning pertaining to
20. The suffix **-gram** refers to a test or procedure that has been ____.
21. Light wood used for airplane models
23. Combining form for the gums
24. Abbreviation for centimeter
25. Suffix meaning vomiting
27. Word root for saliva
28. Where bread is baked.
29. It covers the sun.
30. Suffix meaning visual examination
32. Suffix meaning pertaining to; postal code for Alabama
34. The esophagus is a ___ that connects the mouth with the stomach.
37. An expert knows the __ and outs of a subject.

CROSSWORD PUZZLE UNIT 2: DIGESTIVE SYSTEM

CROSSWORD PUZZLE UNIT 3: URINARY SYSTEM

Across

1. Pain in the urethra
5. Not malignant
8. Opposite of good
10. Suffix for excision
12. The suffix **-stomy** means ____ a new opening.
14. Adenoma is the medical term for a ___ of a gland.
16. Exists
17. Ceremony or ritual, such as a wedding
19. Abbreviation for intravenous pyelogram
20. A Houston football player
22. Shakespeare'a play: ___ *Ado About Nothing*
24. Combining form for hardening
28. Incision of the renal pelvis
31. Poisonous substances in the urine
32. The medical term renogastric means pertaining to the kidney and ____.
33. Impersonal pronoun, or what's not over 'til the fat lady sings.
34. Suffix meaning abnormal condition
36. The medical term for herniation of the rectum
38. Meaning of the suffix **-pathy**
39. Crushing a of stone or calculus

Down

1. Combining form for ureter
2. Medical word root for intestine
3. Medical word root for blood
4. The coiled capillaries in the nephron
5. Hematuria is the medical term for____ in the urine.
6. Suffix meaning inflammation
7. Nocturia means urination during the _____.
9. Conditional word
11. _____ disease is an illness marked by inflammation of the glomeruli.
13. Not important; legally, not adult
15. Suffix meaning involuntary contraction
18. Word root for the ileum
21. Combining form meaning white
22. The southern neighbor of Texas
23. Incontinence is the medical term for loss of ____ of urination.
25. Combining form for the bladder
26. Suffix meaning tumor
27. Suffix meaning suture
28. Suffix meaning prolapse
29. Rocky's favorite greeting: "_, Adrian!"
30. **Aden/o** refers to a _____.
33. Marilyn Monroe movie: *The Seven Year __*.
35. Feminine pronoun
37. To perform a nephrotomy is to __ into a kidney.
38. Extrasensory perception

CROSSWORD PUZZLE UNIT 3: URINARY SYSTEM

CROSSWORD PUZZLE UNIT 4: INTEGUMENTARY SYSTEM

Across

1. A physician who specializes in diseases of the skin
6. "____ and stones may break my bones."
9. Opposite of subtract
10. Mary's wooly pet
11. Condition of inflammation of a sinus
12. The suffix **-oma** denotes a ____.
15. Number of letters in the alphabet
19. A condition of hardening
21. **Tox/o** and **toxic/o** are both combining forms that denote ____.
23. Decrease in the number of cells
26. Opposite of south
27. ". . . at the ___ of a hat."
28. The suffix that means swallow, or eat
29. The condition of softening of the nails.

Down

1. _____ mellitus is a disorder caused by the inability of the body to produce or use insulin.
2. **Erythr/o** is the combining form for this color.
3. Prefix meaning self
4. Suffix meaning abnormal condition
5. Suffix that means inflammation
7. Abnormal condition of blueness
8. Prefix meaning under
13. Literally, "black tumor"; a dark mole or tumor
14. Prefix meaning above or upon.
16. Abbreviation for white blood count
17. Forty winks
18. Literally, "yellow tumor"
20. Bashful
22. The word root that means fat is ___.
24. Prefix meaning many
25. The building block of matter
26. **Onych/o** is the combining form denoting ___.

CROSSWORD PUZZLE UNIT 4: INTEGUMENTARY SYSTEM

CROSSWORD PUZZLE UNIT 5: REPRODUCTIVE SYSTEM

Across

1. Cowper's glands are also known as the _____ glands.
5. The two combining forms for vagina are **vagin/o** and ____.
8. The word root for bladder or sac is __.
10. The word root for fallopian tube (oviduct) is ____.
12. The combining form for birth is __.
15. The suffix **-oma** denotes a ____.
16. Gynecology is the study of the reproductive system of ___.
18. Hormone produced in the testes
19. Personal pronoun
20. Suffix meaning specialist in the study of
21. Condition in which there is a lack of sperm
25. Prefix meaning after
26. The combining form **cervic/o** de- notes both the neck and the ___ uteri.
29. Air pollution
31. Baseball legend ___ Berra
33. Host country for 1992 Olympic Summer Games
37. Combining form for breast
38. Excision of a prostate gland

Down

1. **Mast/o** is the combining form for _____.
2. One of the combining forms for testicle
3. What to do when you are hungry
4. Medical word that literally means blood tumor.
6. Inflamed condition of the ovary
7. The uterus is the ___ that nourishes the embryo.
9. The suffix meaning instrument to cut is __.
10. A facelift is considered a form of plastic _____.
11. Abnormal tissue developments
13. Melodies
14. John, Paul, George, and Ringo
17. The oviducts transport ___ from ovaries to uterus.
22. Suffix meaning fixation __
23. Suffix meaning enlargement ____.
24. Suffix meaning involuntary contraction or twitching ___.
27. Combining form for the vas deferens
28. Ten cents; one thin __
30. Combining form for mucus
32. Suffix meaning tumor _
34. Postal code for Pennsylvania
35. Michael Jackson hit *Beat* _.
36. Opposite of yes

CROSSWORD PUZZLE UNIT 5: REPRODUCTIVE SYSTEM

CROSSWORD PUZZLE UNIT 6: RESPIRATORY SYSTEM

Across

1. The medical term for nostrils (plural)
4. Dilation of the bronchi
8. The combining form for fungus
10. The combining form denoting straight
11. The word root for lung or air is ___.
14. The trachea divides into __ branches, called bronchi.
16. A physician uses a laryngoscope to visually _____ a patient's larynx.
18. The medical term for swallowing air is _____.
20. Past tense of sit
21. Most broad
23. Medical term for involuntary contractions (plural)
24. Word root for mouth
25. Suffix meaning disease
26. Another word for spasms
29. Suffix meaning inflammation
31. The suffix **-oma** means ___.
32. Medical term meaning pertaining to the lobe
34. Combining form for teeth
35. 30, 31, or 28 days
37. Surgical repair of the throat
38. Combining form for blood

Down

1. Inflammation of the nose
2. The combining form for nose
3. The suffix **-rrhaphy** means ___.
4. Slang for weak or bad; "He has a __ knee."
5. New formation or growth.
6. Pertaining to the chest
7. Suffix meaning instrument to view
9. Prefix meaning good
12. Opposite of enter
13. Postal code for Maine
15. Struggling to win a contest
17. The combining form for nose is ___.
18. Respiratory condition marked by wheezing and labored breathing
19. A tumor in the stomach
22. The combining term for windpipe
25. A tumor with a pedicle (stem)
27. Suffix that denotes forming a new opening or mouth
28. **or/o** is the combining form for ___.
30. In liquid, bar, or powder form, a substance used to clean
33. Shaft of light
36. Personal pronoun

CROSSWORD PUZZLE UNIT 6: RESPIRATORY SYSTEM

CROSSWORD PUZZLE UNIT 7: ENDOCRINE AND NERVOUS SYSTEMS

Across

1. Absence of speech
4. The _____ gland is an endocrine gland located in the brain.
6. Combining form denoting sweat
9. Inflammation of the spinal cord
10. Entertained
12. Combining form for front
13. Combining forms for the testes: _____/ and **orchid/o**
16. Abbreviation for posteroanterior
18. Number of players on a baseball team
19. The medical word for blood clot is _____.
21. The prefix meaning excessive is ___.
23. Military order: "_ ease!"
25. Cerebroid means _____ cerebrum.
28. Suffix meaning flow or discharge
29. The suffix **-phasia** means ___.
31. Combining form for mouth
32. Ice T's style of music
35. Combining form for the skin
36. An endocrine gland, located in the upper mediastinum between the lungs
37. Radiology is the _____of x-rays and radioactive substances.

Down

1. Combining form denoting a gland
2. Word root for blood
3. Source of vitamin C: citric __
4. Toxicology is the study of _____.
5. Mother's sister
6. Bursting forth of blood
7. Prefix for difficult
8. Suffix that means resembling
10. Postal code for President Clinton's home state
11. Second sight
12. Hypocalcemia is an _____ low blood calcium level.
14. Combining form for cerebrum (brain)
15. Noun suffix meaning condition
17. Combining form for the extremities
19. Endocrine gland in the neck
20. Cerebral _____ is partial paralysis and muscular incoordination caused by damage to the cerebrum before or during birth.
22. Suffix for disease
24. A waiter's reward
25. Combining form for radiation
26. Opposite of long
27. Word root for nerve
30. **Radi/o** is the combining form for radiation or ___.
33. __ *the World Turns*
34. Abbreviation for physical therapist

CROSSWORD PUZZLE UNIT 7: ENDOCRINE AND NERVOUS SYSTEMS

CROSSWORD PUZZLE UNIT 8: MUSCULOSKELETAL SYSTEM

Across

1. Instrument to measure the head
5. Osteomalacia caused by vitamin deficiency
8. Combining form for spinal cord or bone marrow
9. To cut the hair or nails
11. Suffix meaning cell
12. Shiny metal disk for decorating clothes
15. Ma's mate
16. Pertaining to the lower back and sacrum
20. Suffix meaning surgical repair
21. Combining form for the skull
22. Root word for cell
23. A chondrocyte is a cartilage _____.
26. Suffix meaning blood
27. Combining form for liver
30. Prefix meaning around
31. Combining form for joint
33. Pertaining to the side
34. Disease of the meninges

Down

1. Combining form for calcium
2. Upper arm bone
3. Combining form for muscle
4. Pertaining to the chest
6. Suffix meaning inflammation
7. Combining form meaning vertebra
9. The coccyx is the ___ of the vertebral column.
10. Postal code for Maine
13. Prefix meaning four
14. Myelomalacia means softening of the spinal __.
15. Out of the frying __ into the fire.
17. The year before 1 A.D. was 1 _._.
18. Abbrev. for South America
19. Root word for x-ray
22. Wrist bone
24. Combining form for blood
25. **Spondyl/o** is the combining form for _ _.
27. Calcaneum is the medical term for the ____.
28. What Jack Horner found in his pie.
29. Suffix meaning incision
32. The Boston __ Party

CROSSWORD PUZZLE UNIT 8: MUSCULOSKELETAL SYSTEM

CROSSWORD PUZZLE UNIT 9: CARDIOVASCULAR AND LYMPHATIC SYSTEMS

Across

1. Narrowing or stricture of the aorta
5. Word root for blood clot
8. Rapid breathing
10. Not easy
11. Hemangioma is a ___ of a blood vessel.
12. Arteriorrhaphy is the suture of an ____.
14. Abbreviation for interatrial septum
18. Muscular middle layer of the heart
20. Abbreviation for sinoatrial
22. Dilation or ballooning of the wall of an artery
23. Postal code for Indiana
26. Wild cat with tufted ears
27. Abbreviation for Social Security
29. Combining form for vein
32. Abbreviation for atrioventricular
33. IVC is the abbreviation for inferior vena __.
34. Abbreviation for myocardial infarct
35. Medical term for fainting
36. The bicuspid valve between the left atrium and left ventricle is the ____ valve.
37. Suture of the heart

Down

1. Combining form for artery
2. What red blood cells pick up in the lungs
3. The night before a holiday
4. Pertaining to the groin
5. Pertaining to the chest
6. The ___ pulmonary arteries pump blood to the lungs.
7. Prefix meaning slow
9. Word root for dead or death
10. Opposite of from
13. Powder for violin bows and baseballs
15. Medical term for a cavity
16. Tumor in the lymphatic system
17. Opposite of departure
18. Feminist magazine or postal code for Mississippi
19. Suffix meaning softening
21. Apprehension or worry
24. Suffix meaning involuntary contraction
25. Word root for blood
28. Mark left in the skin by wound healing
30. Prefix for two
31. Word root for muscle
35. Sidney Poitier movie: *To __, With Love*

CROSSWORD PUZZLE UNIT 9: CARDIOVASCULAR AND LYMPHATIC SYSTEMS

CROSSWORD PUZZLE UNIT 10: THE SPECIAL SENSES

Across

1. Disease of the choroid
6. Small, stirrup-shaped bone in the middle ear
10. Slang for all right; book title: *I'm __, You're __*
11. Half dozen
13. Name for the noisiest rock music: heavy __
14. Structure that filters lymph
16. Combining form for the eustachian tube
17. Ma's mate
18. Opposite of down
21. Social insect
22. Excision of all or part of the eyelid
26. Jazz singer __ Fitzgerald
27. Otalgias
29. Jailbreaks; vacations
31. Word root for eye
34. Medical term for incision
36. The suffixes **-algia** and **-dynia** denote _ _.
38. Suffix meaning the study of
39. Innermost of the three layers of the eye
40. Rupture of the cornea

Down

1. Transparent membrane at the front of the eye
2. Word root for ear
3. Suffix meaning inflammation
4. The outer ear
5. John Lennon' widow
6. Abbreviation for sinoatrial
7. Word root for eardrum
8. Suffix meaning disease
9. The white of the eye
12. Condition in which objects appear yellow
15. Diplopia is a condition of ____ vision.
17. List of employees to be paid
19. Suffix meaning surgical repair
20. A faun's mother
23. Spiral tube in the inner ear
24. Postal code for Massachusetts
25. **Pharyng/o** is the combining form for _ ___.
26. Word root for red
28. Complete the word: Involuntary contractions of the eyelid are blepharo ___.
30. Male offspring
32. Combining form for blood
33. Tree-killing pest: Gypsy ___.
35. Thin cushion
37. Writing fluid

CROSSWORD PUZZLE UNIT 10: SPECIAL SENSES

CROSSWORD PUZZLE SOLUTIONS, UNIT 2: DIGESIVE SYSTEM

[1]E	S	[2]O	P	[3]H	A	[4]G	O	T	[5]O	M	[6]E		[7]G	A	S	[8]T	R	I	[9]C
N		R		E		L			P		Y		I			O			O
[10]T	W	O		P		A		[11]F	E	C	E	[12]S			[13]E	X	C	E	L
E			[14]P	A	I	N			N		[15]S	U	B			I			I
R		[16]D		T		D			I			T				[17]C	Y	S	T
[18]O	S	I	S		[19]A	S		[20]R	N		[21]B	U	I	L	D				I
		C			R		[22]B	E	G	[23]G	A	R					[24]C		S
[25]E	C	T	O	M	Y			C		[26]I	L	E	O	[27]S	T	[28]O	M	Y	
M		A				[29]C	R	O	H	N	S			I		V			[30]S
[31]E	N	T	E	R	[32]A	L		R		[33]G	A	[34]T		A		E			C
S		I			[35]L	O	U	D		I		U		[36]L	[37]I	N	G	U	O
I		N				U		E		V		B			N				P
[38]S	I	G	M	O	I	D		[39]D	U	O	D	E	N	O	S	T	O	M	Y

CROSSWORD PUZZLE SOLUTIONS, UNIT 3: URINARY SYSTEM

[1]U	R	[2]E	T	[3]H	R	A	L	[4]G	I	A				[5]B	E	N	[6]I	G	[7]N
R		N		E				L			[8]E	V	[9]I	L			T		I
[10]E	C	T	O	M	Y			O		[11]B			[12]F	O	R	[13]M	I	N	G
T		E		A		[14]T	U	M	O	R		[15]S		O		[16]I	S		H
E		[17]R	[18]I	T	E			E		[19]I	V	P		D		N			T
R			L					R		G		A				O			
[20]O	I	[21]L	E	R			[22]M	U	[23]C	H		[24]S	[25]C	L	E	R	[26]O		[27]R
		E			[28]P	[29]Y	E	L	O	T	O	M	Y				M		R
[30]G		[31]U	R	O	T	O	X	I	N	S			[32]S	T	O	M	A	C	H
L		K			O		I		T			[33]I	T						A
A		[34]O	[35]S	I	S		C		[36]R	E	C	T	O	[37]C	E	L	[38]E		P
N			H		I		O		O			C		U			S		H
[38]D	I	S	E	A	S	E			[39]L	I	T	H	O	T	R	I	P	S	Y

CROSSWORD PUZZLE SOLUTIONS, UNIT 4: INTEGUMENTARY SYSTEM

[1]D	E	[2]R	M	[3]A	T	[4]O	L	O	G	[5]I	S	T		[6]S	T	I	[7]C	K	[8]S
I		E		U		S				T							Y		U
[9]A	D	D		T		I				I						[10]L	A	M	B
B				O		[11]S	I	N	U	S	I	T	I	S			N		
E																	O		
[12]T	U	[13]M	O	R	S		[14]E				[15]T	[16]W	E	[17]N	T	Y	S	I	[18]X
E		E					P					B		A			I		A
[19]S	C	L	E	R	O	[20]S	I	S				C		[21]P	O	I	S	O	N
		A				H													T
[22]A		N			[23]C	Y	T	O	[24]P	E	N	I	[25]A		[26]N	O	R	T	H
[27]D	R	O	P						O				T		A				O
I		M							L				O		I				M
[28]P	H	A	G	I	A		[29]O	N	Y	C	H	O	M	A	L	A	C	I	A

CROSSWORD PUZZLE SOLUTIONS, UNIT 5: REPRODUCTIVE SYSTEM

Completed crossword solution grid (letters as filled in; numbered starting cells shown with their clue numbers, black squares shown as ■):

¹B	R	E	A	S	¹⁸T	■	²⁴S	²⁵P	A	³³S	³⁷M	
U	■	¹¹D	Y	S	■	²⁰L	A	O	■	I	A	
L	³E	A	S	T	¹⁴B	A	G	S	²⁶C	³⁵I	³⁴P	
⁴H	E	M	A	¹⁵T	O	I	T	²⁷V	E	R	³⁶N	³⁸P
R	A	L	¹³T	U	⁹T	O	M	²²P	S	E	I	R
⁵C	A	L	P	O	¹⁶W	O	R	¹⁹M	E	I	S	O
⁶O	O	L	P	H	O	R	G	¹⁷E	G	G	I	S
⁷O	R	G	A	N	■	■	²³M	E	G	A	L	Y
P	■	I	N	■	E	G	S	■	³⁰M	O	U	C
L	O	■	¹⁰S	U	R	G	E	²⁹S	S	U	²⁸D	T
³¹Y	³²O	M	M	A	E	R	M	²¹A	¹²N	⁸C	I	O
²O	R	⁸C	H	I	O	■	■	X	G	Y	M	M

CROSSWORD PUZZLE SOLUTIONS, UNIT 6: RESPIRATORY SYSTEM

[1]N	A	[2]R	E	[3]S		[4]B	R	O	[5]N	C	H	I	E	C	[6]T	A	S	I	[7]S
A		H		U		U			E						H				C
S		I		T		[8]M	Y	C	O			[9]E			[10]O	R	T	H	O
I		N		U					[11]P	N	[12]E	U	[13]M		R				P
[14]T	W	O		R		[15]C			L		X		[16]E	X	A	M	I	[17]N	E
I			[18]A	E	R	O	P	H	A	[19]G	I	A			C			A	
S			S			M			[20]S	A	T			[21]W	I	D	E	S	[22]T
			T		[23]S	P	A	S	M	S					C			[24]O	R
[25]P	A	T	H	Y		E				[26]T	I	C	[27]S			[28]M			A
O			M		[29]I	T	I	[30]S		R			[31]T	U	M	O	R		C
[32]L	O	B	A	[33]R		I		[34]O	D	O	N	T	O			U			H
Y				A		N		A		M			[35]M	O	N	T	[36]H		E
[37]P	H	A	R	Y	N	G	O	P	L	A	S	T	Y			[38]H	E	M	O

CROSSWORD PUZZLE SOLUTIONS, UNIT 7: ENDOCRINE AND NERVOUS SYSTEMS

CROSSWORD PUZZLE SOLUTIONS, UNIT 8: MUSCULOSKELETAL SYSTEM

Completed crossword solution grid (letters shown with their clue numbers where numbered; ■ = blocked cell):

¹C	²H	³M	⁴T	⁵R	⁶I	⁷S	⁸M	⁹T	¹⁰M	¹¹C	¹²S	¹³Q	¹⁴C
¹⁵P	¹⁶L	¹⁷B	¹⁸S	¹⁹R	²⁰P	²¹C	²²C	²³C	²⁴H	²⁵S	²⁶E	²⁷H	²⁸P
²⁹T	³⁰P	³¹A	³²T	³³L	³⁴M								

Grid letters (as filled in the solution), read with the page rotated:

- SPONDYLO… / …ROMY
- RHEUMATOID / ARTHROPATHY
- CALCANEUS
- MYELOGRAM
- CLAVICLE
- THORACIC
- STERNUM
- QUADRICEPS
- CARPAL
- PLASTER
- HEEL

CROSSWORD PUZZLE SOLUTIONS, UNIT 9: CARDIOVASCULAR AND LYMPHATIC SYSTEMS

1A	O	R	T	2O	S	T	3E	N	O	S	4I	S			5T	H	6R	O	M	7B
R				X			V				N				H		I			R
8T	A	C	H	Y	P	9N	E	A			G		10T	O	U	G	H			A
E				G		E				11T	U	M	O	R			H			D
R				E		C				I			12A	R	T	E		13R	Y	
14I	A	15S		N		R		16L		N			C					O		
O		I			17A		18M	Y	O	C	A	R	D	I	U	19M		20S	21A	
	22A	N	E	U	R	Y	S	M			L		C		A			23I	N	
24S		U		R			P		25H							26L	Y	N	X	
P		27S	28S	I		29P	H	L	E	30B	O		31M		A				I	
32A	V			33C	A	V	A		34M	I		35S	Y	N	C	O	P	E	
S			A		A		O					I			I			T	
36M	I	T	R	A	L		37C	A	R	D	I	O	R	R	H	A	P	H	Y

ANATOMY COLORING ACTIVITIES

A coloring activity is included for each unit to reinforce the anatomy of the body system. The coloring instructions are summarized here. Review this information, as well as the entire illustration, before you begin; use colored pencils.

As a general rule, use light colors for the larger areas, and dark colors for the smaller areas. Color in the order given on each page. Do not use the same color for two consecutive organs. Begin by coloring the part of the drawing marked "a." In the first illustration, The Digestive System (page 189), this is the oral cavity.

Anatomy Activity: Unit 2, The Digestive System

To complete this activity, read the instructions on page 188.   Begin by coloring the part of the drawing marked "a."   This is the oral cavity.

The digestive system.

ALIMENTARY TRACT
Oral cavity **a**
Pharynx **b**
Esophagus **c**
Stomach **d**
Small Intestine:
    Duodenum **e**
    Jejunum **f**
    Ileum **g**
Large Intestine:
    Appendix **h**
    Ascending colon **i**
    Transverse colon **j**
    Descending colon **k**
    Sigmoid colon **l**
    Rectum **m**
    Anal canal **n**

ACCESSORY ORGANS
Teeth **o**
Tongue **p**
Salivary Glands:
    Sublingual **q**
    Submaxillary **r**
    Parotid **s**
Liver **t**
Gallbladder **u**
Common bile duct **v**
Pancreas **w**
Spleen **x**

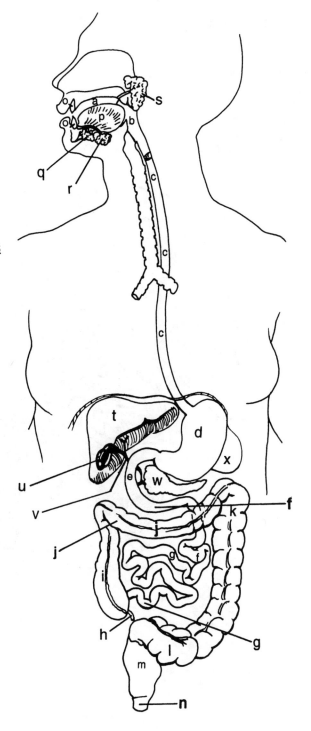

Anatomy Activity: Unit 2, Accessory Organs of Digestion

To complete this activity, read the instructions on page 188. Begin by coloring the part of the drawing marked "a." This is the liver.

Anterior view of the accessory organs of digestion: the liver, gall bladder, and pancreas. (Adapted from Gylys, BA and Wedding, ME: Medical Terminology: A Systems Approach, ed 2. FA Davis, Philadelphia, 1988, p 94.)

Liver **a**
Gallbladder **b**
Pancreas **c**
Hepatic duct **d**
Cystic duct **e**
Pancreatic duct **f**
Common bile duct **g**
Duodenum **h**

Anatomy Activity: Unit 3 Urinary System

To complete this activity, read the instructions on page 188. Begin by coloring the part of the drawing marked "a." This is the kidney.

The urinary system. (Adapted from Gylys, BA and Wedding, ME: Medical Terminology: A Systems Approach, ed 2. FA Davis, Philadelphia, 1988, pp 240, 241.)

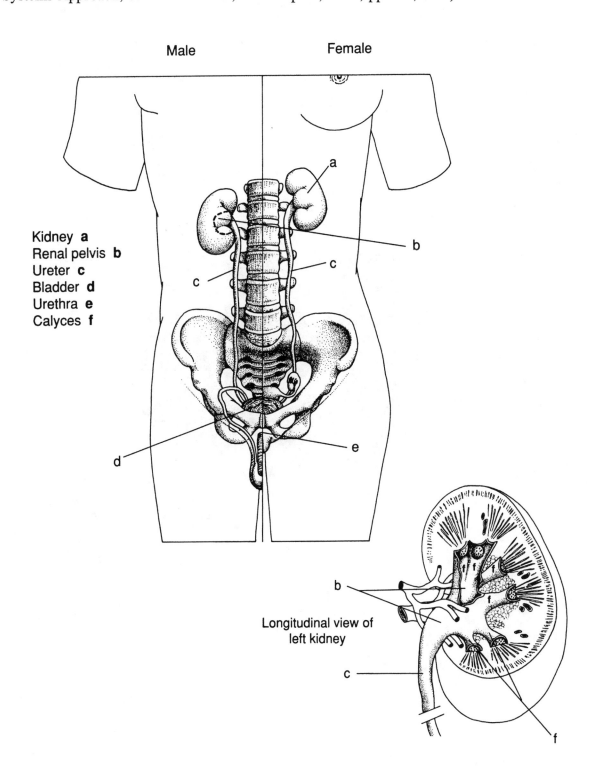

Male   Female

Kidney **a**
Renal pelvis **b**
Ureter **c**
Bladder **d**
Urethra **e**
Calyces **f**

Longitudinal view of
left kidney

Anatomy Activity: Unit 4, Integumentary System

To complete this activity, read the instructions on page 188. Begin by coloring the part of the drawing marked "a." This is the hair shaft.

Cross-section of the skin. (Adapted from Gylys, BA and Wedding, ME: Medical Terminology. A Systems Approach, ed 2. FA Davis, Philadelphia, 1988, p 66.)

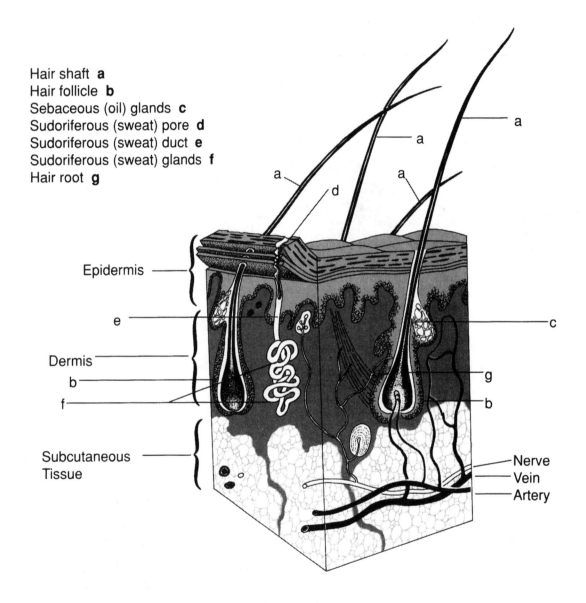

Hair shaft **a**
Hair follicle **b**
Sebaceous (oil) glands **c**
Sudoriferous (sweat) pore **d**
Sudoriferous (sweat) duct **e**
Sudoriferous (sweat) glands **f**
Hair root **g**

Epidermis

e

Dermis

b

f

Subcutaneous
Tissue

a

a

a

a

d

c

g

b

Nerve
Vein
Artery

Anatomy Activity: Unit 5, Female Reproductive System

To complete this activity, read the instructions on page 188. Begin by coloring the part of the drawing marked "a." This is the ovary.

The female reproductive system. (Adapted from Gylys, BA and Wedding, ME: Medical Terminology: A Systems Approach, ed 2. FA Davis, Philadelphia, 1988, pp 268, 269.)

Internal Reproductive Organs
  Ovary **a**
  Uterine (fallopian) tube **b**
  Uterus **c**
  Vagina **d**

External Structures of Vagina
  Labia minora **e**
  Labia majora **f**
  Clitoris **g**
  Bartholin's gland **h**

Other Structures
  Cervix (neck of uterus) **i**
  Bladder (Urinary System) **j**
  Rectum (Gastrointestinal System) **k**
  Anus (Gastrointestinal System) **l**
  Urethra (Urinary System) **m**

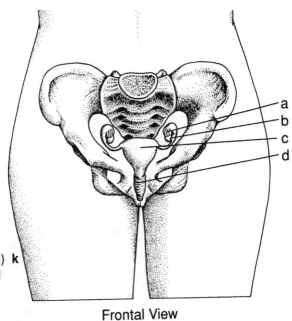

Frontal View

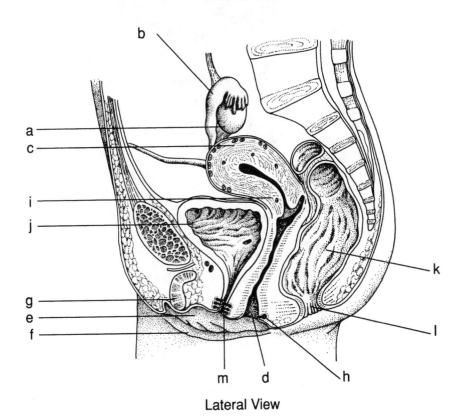

Lateral View

Anatomy Activity: Unit 5, Male Reproductive System

To complete this activity, read the instructions on page 188. Begin by coloring the part of the drawing marked "a." This is the testis.

The male reproductive system. (Adapted from Gylys, BA and Wedding, ME: Medical Terminology: A Systems Approach, ed 2. FA Davis, Philadelphia, 1988, p 244.)

Male Reproductive Organs
  Testis **a**
  Scrotum **b**
  Epididymis **c**
  Vas deferens **d**
  Seminal vesicle **e**
  Prostate gland **f**
  Cowper's (Bulbourethral) gland **g**
  Penis **h**
  Glans penis **i**

Other Structures
  Bladder (Urinary System) **j**
  Urethra (Urinary System) **k**

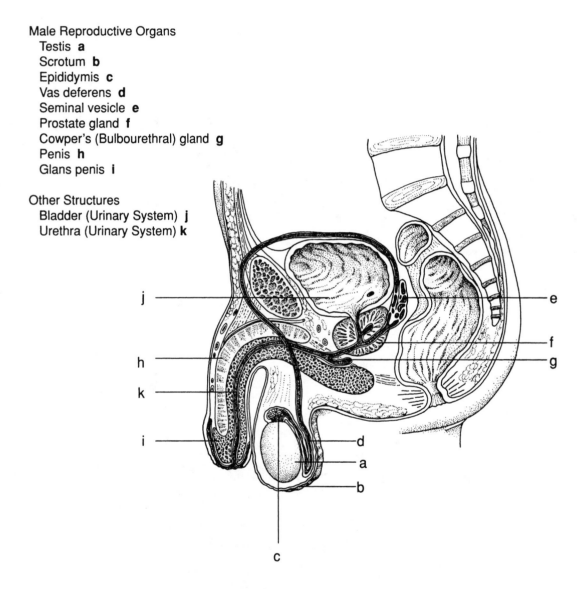

Anatomy Activity: Unit 6, The Respiratory System

To complete this activity, read the instructions on page 188. Begin by coloring the part of the drawing marked "a." This is the nasal cavity.

Use red for the venule (I), which returns oxygenated blood to the heart from the alveolus. Use blue for the arteriole(j), which carries blood to capillaries. Use purple for the capillary network (k) surrounding the alveolar sac to represent gradual oxygenation.

The respiratory system. (Adapted from Gylys, BA and Wedding, ME: Medical Terminology: A Systems Approach, ed 2. FA Davis, Philadelphia, 1988, p 123.)

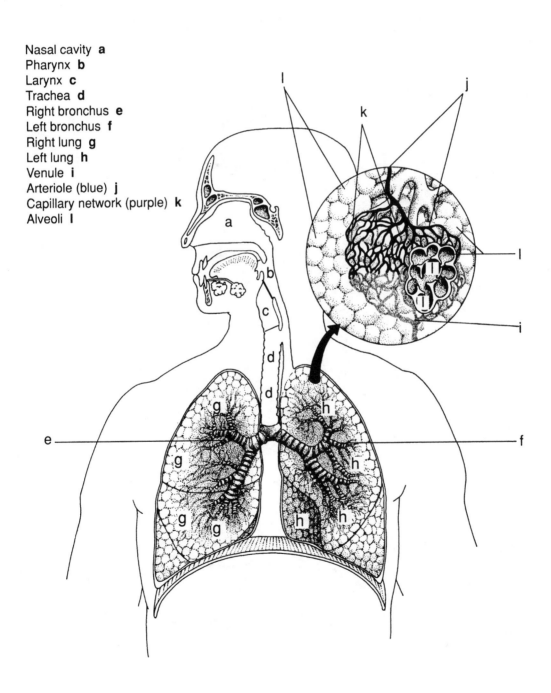

Nasal cavity **a**
Pharynx **b**
Larynx **c**
Trachea **d**
Right bronchus **e**
Left bronchus **f**
Right lung **g**
Left lung **h**
Venule **i**
Arteriole (blue) **j**
Capillary network (purple) **k**
Alveoli **l**

Anatomy Activity: Unit 7, Endocrine and Nervous Systems

To complete this activity, read the instructions on page 188. Begin by coloring the part of the drawing marked "a." This is the pituitary.

Anatomy cavity. (From Gylys, BA and Wedding, ME: Medical Terminology: A Systems Approach, ed 2. FA Davis, Philadelphia, 1988, p 300, with permission.)

Pituitary **a**
Thyroid gland **b**
Pancreas **c**
Adrenal (suprarenal) glands **d**
Parathyroid glands **e**
Pineal gland **f**
Ovary **g**
Testis **h**

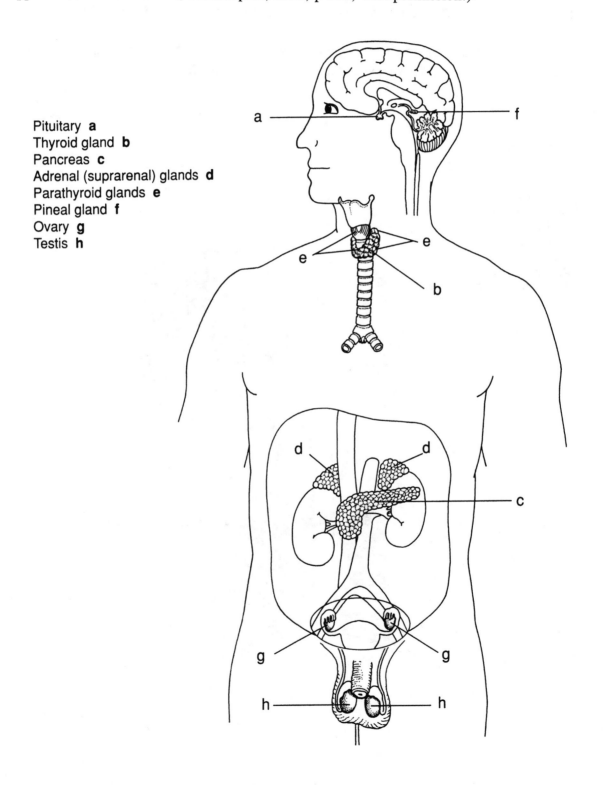

Anatomy Activity: Unit 8, Musculoskeletal System

To complete this activity, read the instructions on page 188. Begin by coloring the part of the drawing marked "a." This is the mandible or lower jaw.

Frontal view of skeleton. (Adapted from Gylys, BA and Wedding, ME: Medical Terminology: A Systems Approach, ed 2. FA Davis, Philadelphia, 1988, p 204.)

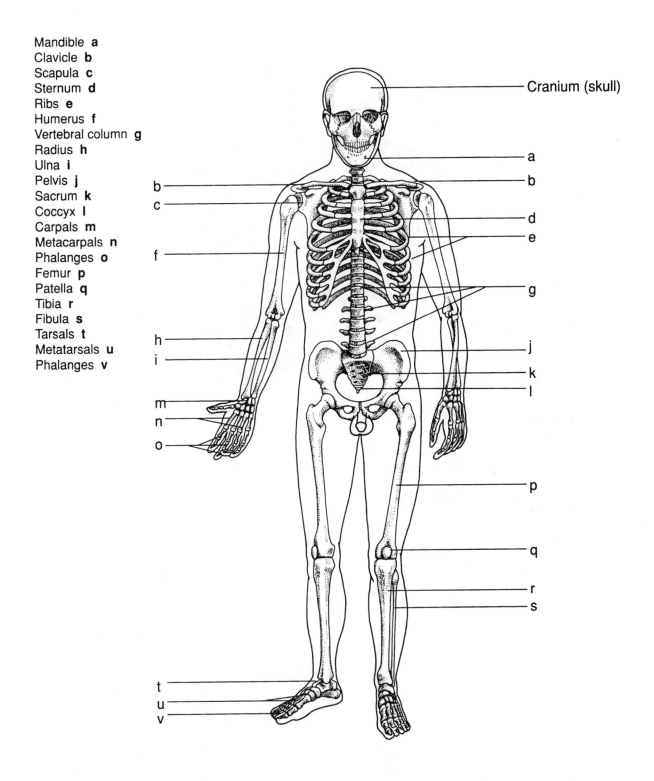

Mandible **a**
Clavicle **b**
Scapula **c**
Sternum **d**
Ribs **e**
Humerus **f**
Vertebral column **g**
Radius **h**
Ulna **i**
Pelvis **j**
Sacrum **k**
Coccyx **l**
Carpals **m**
Metacarpals **n**
Phalanges **o**
Femur **p**
Patella **q**
Tibia **r**
Fibula **s**
Tarsals **t**
Metatarsals **u**
Phalanges **v**

Cranium (skull)

Anatomy Activity: Unit 9, Cardiovascular and Lymphatic Systems

To complete this activity, read the instructions on page 188. Begin by coloring the part of the drawing marked "a." This is the aorta and its three branches.

Anatomy activity. (Adapted from Gylys, BA and Wedding, ME: Medical Terminology: A Systems Approach, ed 2. FA Davis, Philadelphia, 1988, p 149.)

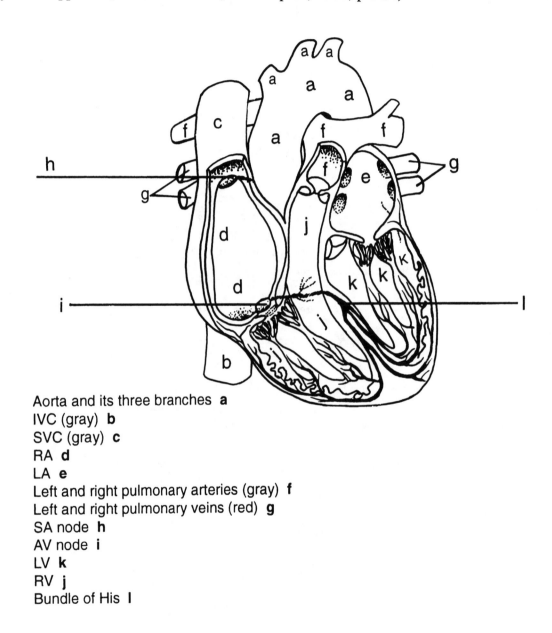

Aorta and its three branches **a**
IVC (gray) **b**
SVC (gray) **c**
RA **d**
LA **e**
Left and right pulmonary arteries (gray) **f**
Left and right pulmonary veins (red) **g**
SA node **h**
AV node **i**
LV **k**
RV **j**
Bundle of His **l**

Anatomy Activity: Unit 10, Special Senses: Anterior View Of The Eye

To complete this activity, read the instructions on page 188. Begin by coloring the part of the drawing marked "a." This is the pupil.

The anterior view of the eye. (Adapted from Gylys, BA and Wedding, ME: Medical Terminology: A Systems Approach, ed 2. FA Davis, Philadelphia, 1988, p 354.)

Pupil (black) **a**
iris (brown) **b**
Sclera (white) **c**
Lacrimal sac and nasolacrimal duct (blue) **d**
Lacrimal glands (blue) **e**
Eyelid **f**

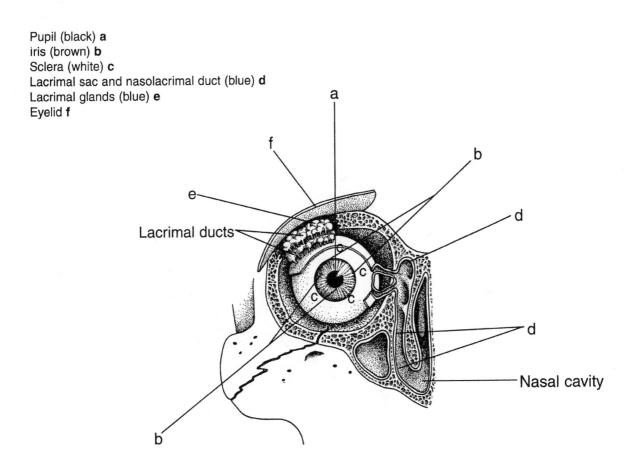

Anatomy Activity: Unit 10, Special Senses: External, Middle, and Inner Ear

To complete this activity, read the instructions on page 188. Begin by coloring the part of the drawing marked "a." This is the auricle. Color the auricle (a) and ear canal (b) the same color.

Anatomy of the external, middle, and inner ear. (Adapted from Gylys, BA and Wedding, ME: Medical Terminology: A Systems Approach, ed 2. FA Davis, Philadelphia, 1988, p 353.)

Auricle **a**
Ear canal **b**
Tympanic membrane **c**
Malleus **d**
Incus **e**
Stapes (set in oval window) **f**
Eustachian (auditory) tube **g**
Cochlea **h**
Semicircular canals **i**
Vestibule **j**

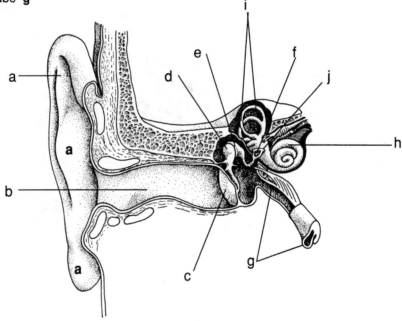

INSTRUCTIONAL AIDS

Audiocassette Tapes

Included in each book are two standard 90-minute audiocassette tapes that are designed to strengthen the student's spelling, pronunciation, and knowledge of the meaning of medical terms. An audiocassette exercise in each unit provides continuous reinforcement of correct usage of medical terms, so this skill is adequately developed for entry-level positions in the health-care industry.

The **audiocassette tape** directs the student to look at the word on the audiocassette list for the particular unit being covered and to listen to the pronunciation and definition of each word, saying the term aloud as it is dictated. A self-tutorial spelling exercise is also integrated for each unit on the tape.

The **audiocassette tape** can also be used on a standard cassette transcriber for beginning transcription courses. This feature permits medical secretarial and medical transcription students to learn beginning transcription skills by typing each word as they hear it pronounced. After the words are typed, the spelling can be corrected using the audiocassette exercise word list in the textbook.

Assigning specific activities, such as those suggested in the audiocassette exercises, motivates the student to listen to the tapes frequently. They soon recognize that the tapes help them to develop the most basic skill needed in the allied health fields, a knowledge of medical terminology.

Flash Cards

Students can develop flash cards on 3 by 5 index cards for the word elements in a given unit, and these can be used to reinforce retention of the word elements. First, they can compile the cards for the word elements included in the Review section they are completing. Then they can complete and correct the review. If they are not satisfied with their review score, they can study the flash cards again before retaking the review. Have them follow this procedure each time they are ready to complete a review. The flash cards can also be used before they complete the Unit Exercise at the end of each unit.

The flash cards can be labeled according to the unit in which the element was presented and can be organized for study in various ways. The surgical suffixes can be organized in one packet for study purposes. Some flash cards can also be organized according to basic elements (combining forms, suffixes, prefixes) or body systems. Students should be encouraged to use the flash cards for study purposes either in group activities or employed as a self-tutorial approach.

Interactive CD-ROM

The instructor may choose to adopt the book with a multimedia *Interactive Medical Terminology CD-ROM*. This competency-based software is self-paced and includes graphics, voice, a dictionary, help menus, printouts of student's progress, along with numerous activities that are designed at a 90% competency level. The software program supports a self-instructional, competency-based approach to learning, letting students master each task presented before advancing to the next activity. Students work at their own pace in a classroom setting or independently.

Technical Journals

Technical journals are available from public libraries, academic institutions, hospitals, and through the publishers. Direct your students to professional journals for outside assignments. The following is a brief list of some excellent journals:

American Journal of Hematology
Emergency Medicine
Health Care Management Review
Journal of the American Medical Association
Journal of Nursing
Journal of Clinical Endocrinology and Metabolism
New England Journal of Medicine
Nursing Forum
Nutrition and Cancer
Professional Medical Assistant

Many organizations offer educational information to educators. Pamphlets, film strips, and speakers may be available from state and local societies. Check the phone directory under "associations." The following is a brief list of community resources:

American Cancer Society
American Diabetes Association
American Kidney Foundation
American Red Cross
Arthritis Foundation
Lung Association
Multiple Sclerosis Society
Muscular Dystrophy Association
National Hemophilia Foundation

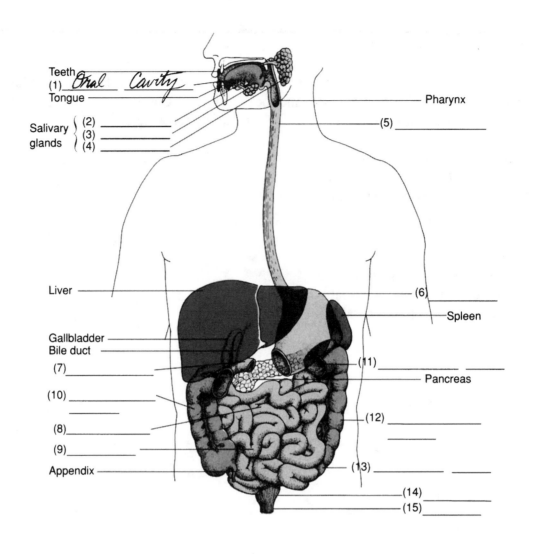

Teeth
(1) _Oral Cavity_
Tongue —————————————————————— Pharynx

Salivary { (2) _____
glands   { (3) _____   (5) _____
         { (4) _____

Liver ——————————————————————— (6) _____

——————————————— Spleen

Gallbladder ———————————
Bile duct ———————————
(7) _____   (11) _____ _____
                         ——————————— Pancreas
(10) _____
     _____   (12) _____
(8) _____   _____
(9) _____
Appendix ———————   (13) _____ _____
                         (14) _____
                         (15) _____

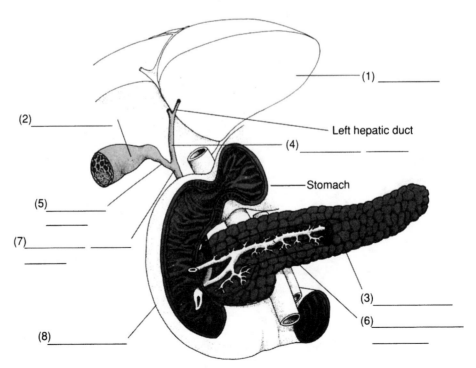

(1) _____

(2) _____   ——————— Left hepatic duct

                         (4) _____ _____

                         ——————— Stomach

(5) _____
    _____

(7) _____
    _____
                         (3) _____
                         (6) _____

(8) _____   _____

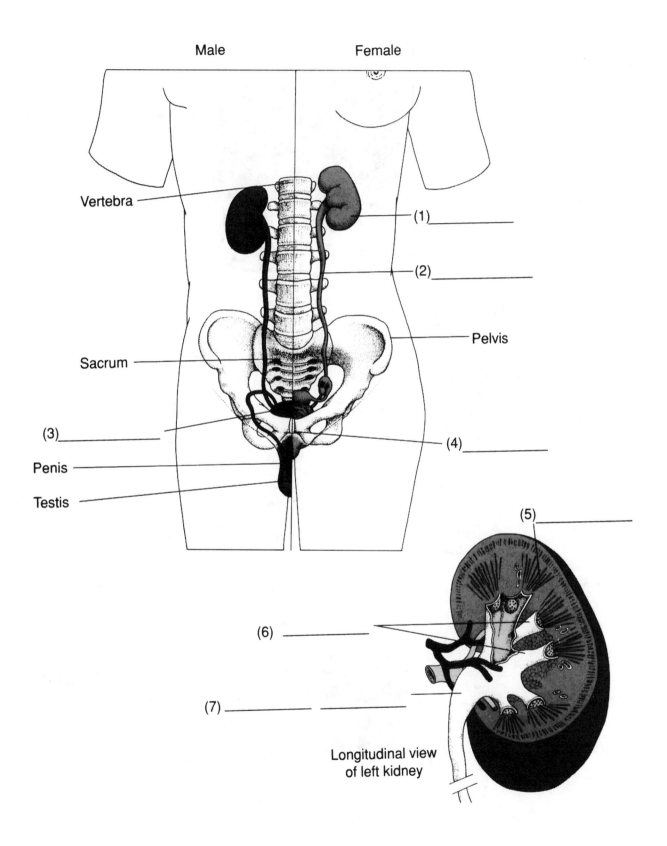

Male   Female

Vertebra

(1)_____

(2)_____

Pelvis

Sacrum

(3)_____

Penis

Testis

(4)_____

(5)_____

(6)_____

(7)_____

Longitudinal view
of left kidney

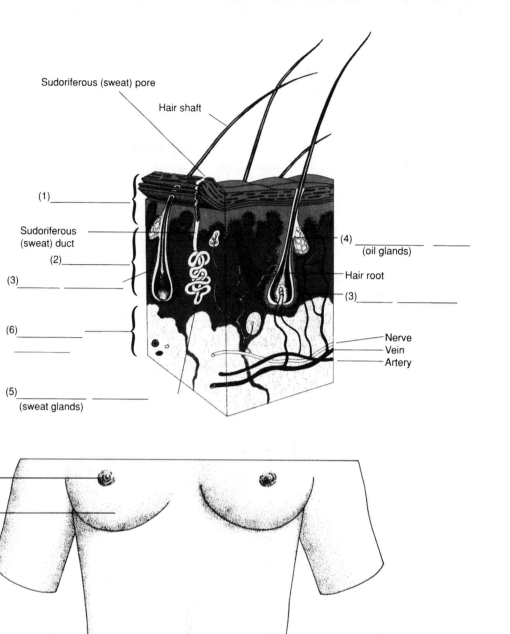

Sudoriferous (sweat) pore

Hair shaft

(1)_____

Sudoriferous (sweat) duct

(2)_____

(3)_____ _____

(6)_____

_____

(5)_____ _____
(sweat glands)

(4)_____ _____
(oil glands)

Hair root

(3)_____ _____

Nerve
Vein
Artery

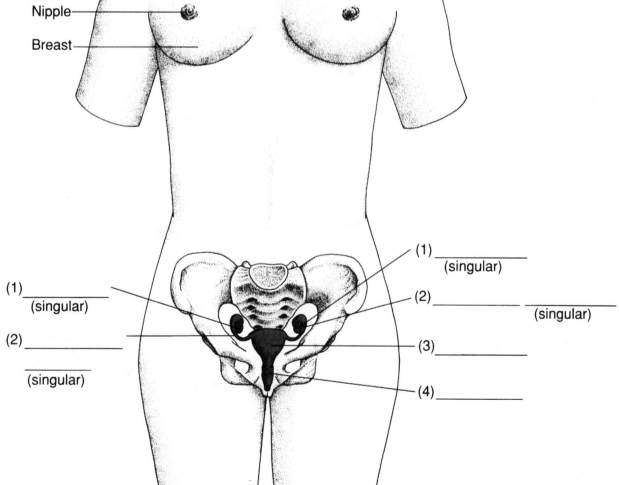

Nipple

Breast

(1)_____
(singular)

(2)_____

_____
(singular)

(1)_____
(singular)

(2)_____ _____
(singular)

(3)_____

(4)_____

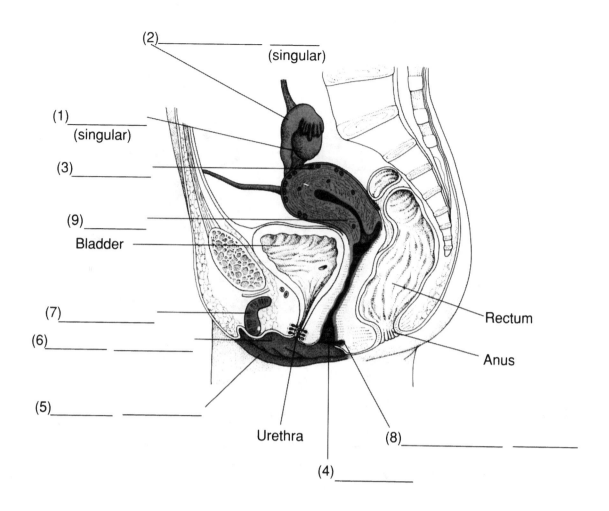

(2)_____ _____
(singular)

(1)_____
(singular)

(3)_____

(9)_____

Bladder _____

(7)_____

(6)_____ _____

(5)_____ _____

Urethra

Rectum

Anus

(8)_____ _____

(4)_____

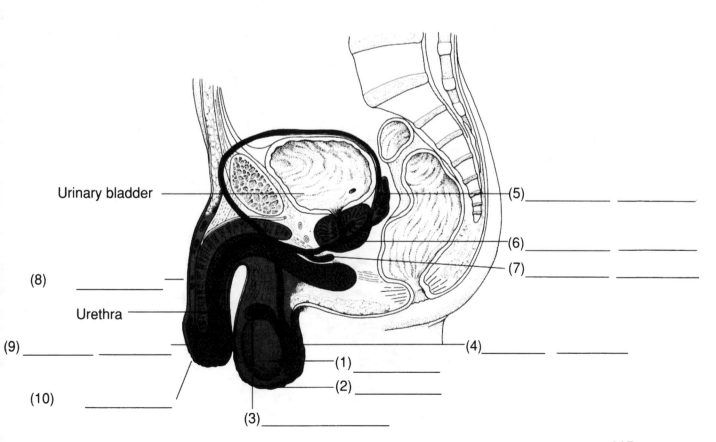

Urinary bladder _____

(8) _____

Urethra

(9) _____ _____

(10) _____

(3)_____

(1) _____

(2) _____

(5)_____ _____

(6)_____ _____

(7)_____ _____

(4)_____ _____

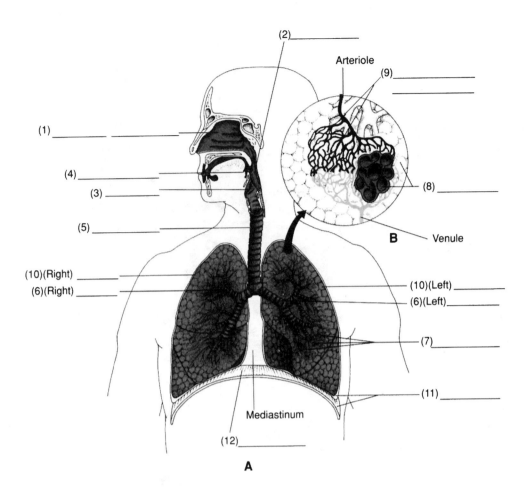

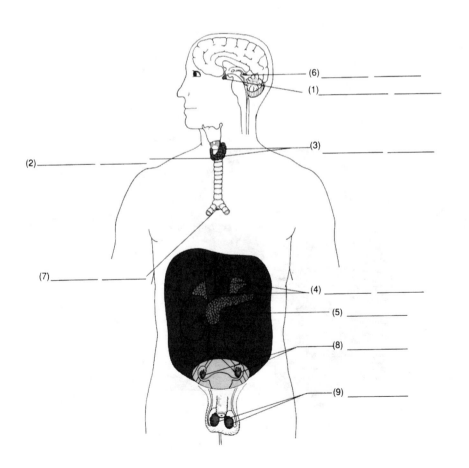

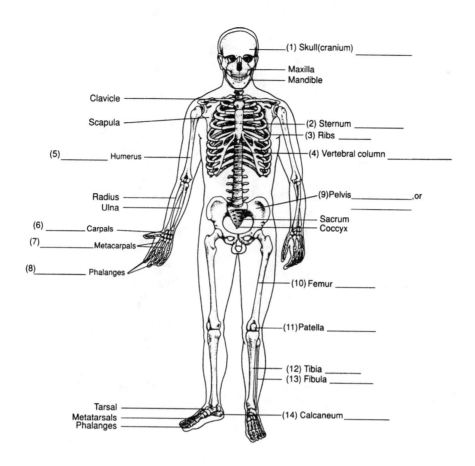

(1) Skull(cranium) _____

Maxilla
Mandible

Clavicle

Scapula

(2) Sternum _____
(3) Ribs _____

(5) _____ Humerus

(4) Vertebral column _____

Radius
Ulna

(9)Pelvis_____,or
_____

Sacrum
Coccyx

(6) _____ Carpals

(7) _____ Metacarpals

(8) _____ Phalanges

(10) Femur _____

(11)Patella _____

(12) Tibia _____
(13) Fibula _____

Tarsal
Metatarsals
Phalanges

(14) Calcaneum_____

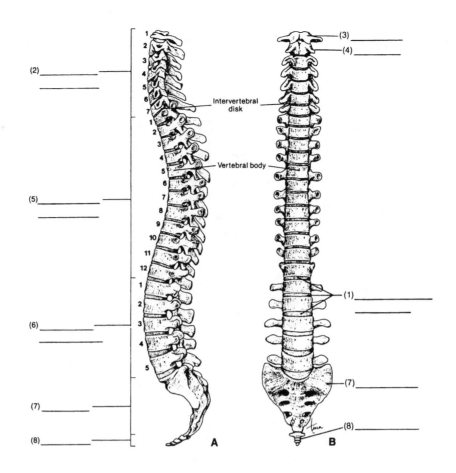

1
2
3
4
5
6
7

Intervertebral disk

1
2
3
4
5
6
7
8
9
10
11
12

Vertebral body

1
2
3
4
5

(2) _____
_____

(5) _____
_____

(6) _____
_____

(7) _____

(8) _____

(3) _____
(4) _____

(1) _____
_____

(7) _____

(8) _____

A   B

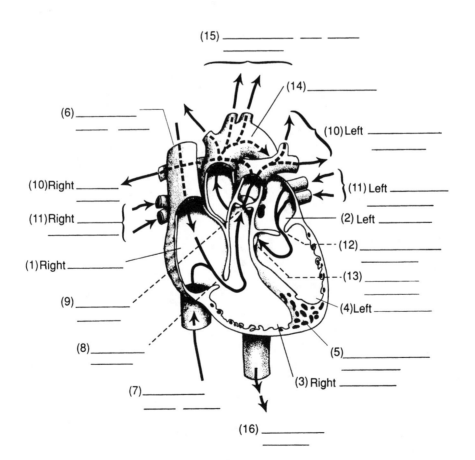

(15) _____ ___ ___

(14) _____

(6) _____
_____

(10) Left _____

(10) Right _____
_____

(11) Left _____

(11) Right _____
_____

(2) Left _____

(12) _____

(1) Right _____

(13) _____

(9) _____
_____

(4) Left _____

(8) _____
_____

(5) _____
_____

(7) _____
___ ___ ___

(3) Right _____

(16) _____
_____

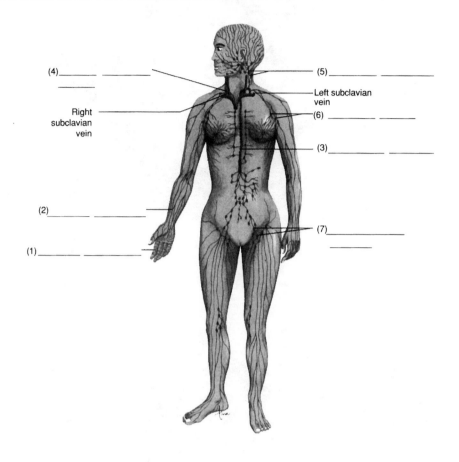

(4)_____ _____

(5)_____ _____

Left subclavian
vein

Right
subclavian
vein

(6) _____ _____

(3)_____ _____

(2)_____ _____

(7)_____

(1)_____ _____

_____

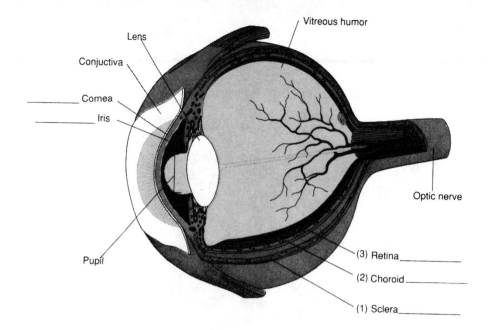

Vitreous humor

Lens

Conjuctiva

Cornea

Iris

Optic nerve

Pupil

(3) Retina_____

(2) Choroid_____

(1) Sclera_____

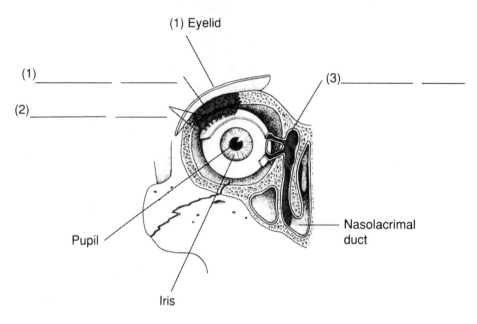

(1) Eyelid

(1)_____ _____

(2)_____ _____

(3)_____ _____

Pupil

Nasolacrimal duct

Iris

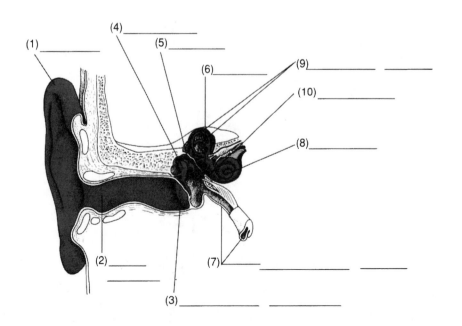

(1)_____

(4)_____

(5)_____

(6)_____

(9)_____ _____

(10)_____

(8)_____

(2)_____

(7)_____ _____ _____

(3)_____ _____

Answer Key for Master Transparencies

UNIT 2 DIGESTIVE SYSTEM
Figure 2–1 Digestive System
1. oral cavity
2. sublingual
3. submaxillary
4. parotid
5. esophagus
6. stomach
7. duodenum
8. jejunum
9. ileum
10. ascending colon
11. transverse colon
12. descending colon
13. sigmoid colon
14. rectum
15. anus

Figure 2–2 Digestive System
1. liver
2. gallbladder
3. pancreas
4. hepatic duct
5. cystic duct
6. common bile ducts
7. duodenum

UNIT 3 URINARY SYSTEM
Figure 3–1 Urinary System
1. kidney
2. ureter
3. bladder
4. urethra
5. nephron
6. calyces
7. renal pelvis

UNIT 4 INTEGUMENTARY SYSTEM
Figure 4–1 Integumentary System
1. epidermis
2. dermis
3. hair follicle
4. sebaceous glands
5. sudoriferous glands
6. subcutaneous tissue

UNIT 5 REPRODUCTIVE SYSTEM
Figures 5–1 and 5–2 Reproductive System
1. ovary
2. fallopian tube
3. uterus
4. vagina
5. labia majora
6. labia minora
7. clitoris
8. Bartholin's glands
9. cervix

Figure 5–3 Reproductive System
1. testis (singular)
2. scrotum
3. epididymis
4. vas deferens
5. seminal vesicles
6. prostate gland
7. Cowper's glands
8. penis
9. glans penis
10. foreskin

UNIT 6 RESPIRATORY SYSTEM
Figure 6–1 Respiratory System
1. nasal cavity
2. pharynx (throat)
3. larynx (voice box)
4. epiglottis
5. trachea (windpipe)
6. bronchus
7. bronchioles
8. alveoli
9. pulmonary capillaries

10. lung
11. pleura
12. diaphragm

UNIT 7 ENDOCRINE AND NERVOUS SYSTEMS

Figure 7-l Endocrine and Nervous Systems

1. pituitary gland
2. thyroid gland
3. parathyroid glands
4. adrenal (suprarenal) glands
5. pancreas
6. pineal gland
7. thymus gland
8. ovaries
9. testes

UNIT 8 MUSCULOSKELETAL SYSTEM

Figure 8-1 Musculoskeletal System

1. crani/o
2. stern/o
3. cost/o
4. vertebr/o
5. humer/o
6. carp/o
7. metacarp/o
8. phalang/o
9. pelv/i, pelv/o
10. femor/o
11. patell/o
12. tibi/o
13. fibul/o
14. calcane/o

Figure 8-3 Musculoskeletal System

1. simple or closed fracture
2. compound or open fracture
3. Greenstick fracture
4. impacted fracture

Figure 8-4 Musculoskeletal System

1. intervertebral disks
2. cervical vertebrae
3. atlas
4. axis

5. thoracic vertebrae
6. lumbar vertebrae
7. sacrum
8. coccyx

UNIT 9 CV AND LYMPHATIC

Figure 9-3 Cardiovascular System

1. right atrium (RA)
2. left atrium (LA)
3. right ventricle (RV)
4. left ventricle (LV)
5. interventricular septum (IVS)
6. superior vena cava (SVC)
7. inferior vena cava (IVC)
8. tricuspid valve
9. pulmonary valve
10. pulmonary arteries
11. pulmonary veins
12. mitral valve
13. aortic valve
14. aorta
15. branches of the aorta
16. descending aorta

Figure 9-5 Cardiovascular System

1. sinoatrial (SA) node
2. RA
3. atrioventricular (AV) node
4. Bundle of His
5. bundle branches
6. Purkinje fibers

Figure 9-8 Lymphatic System

1. lymph capillaries
2. lymph vessels
3. thoracic duct
4. right lymphatic duct
5. cervical nodes
6. axillary nodes
7. inguinal nodes

UNIT 10 SPECIAL SENSES: THE EYES AND EARS
Figure 10–1 Special Senses
1. scler/o
2. choroid/o
3. retin/o
4. kerat/o
5. irid/o
Figure l0-3 Special Senses
1. lacrimal glands
2. lacrimal ducts
3. lacrimal sac
Figure l0-4 Special Senses
1. auricle
2. ear canal
3. tympanic membrane
4. malleus
5. incus
6. stapes
7. eustachian tube
8. cochlea
9. semicircular canals
10. vestibule

6211